TOO BUSY TO GET

Busy

How to Fix Your (Almost) Sexless Relationship

JANE GUYN, PhD RN

Begin to create
your own BEDROOM Blueprint™
https://www.janeguyn.com/startthepath

Disclaimer

The information provided in this book is designed to provide helpful information on the subjects discussed. This book is not meant to be used, nor should it be used, to diagnose or treat any medical condition. For diagnosis or treatment of any medical problem, consult your own physician. Additionally, the book is not meant to be used, nor should it be used to diagnose or treat any psychological condition. For the diagnosis or treatment of any psychological problem, please consult a licensed mental health practitioner. The publisher and author are not responsible for any specific health or mental health needs that may require medical supervision and are not liable for any damages or negative consequences from any treatment, action, application or preparation to any person reading or following the information in this book. References are provided for informational purposes only and do not constitute endorsement of any websites or other sources. Readers should be aware that the websites listed in this book may change.

Praise for

Too Busy to Get Busy

"With the pandemic of the sexless relationship, this book comes along just in time to show couples on the brink of disaster how to find their way. Aiming at the heart of the dilemma, Dr. Jane Guyn helps couples discover a "BEDROOM Blueprint™" that will change their relationship for good."

Dr. Patti Britton, Co-founder of SexCoachU, former AASECT President, author of The Art of Sex Coaching: Transforming Your Practice www.drpattibritton.com

"Jane is a pure delight! Her sincere dedication in supporting couples to find more love, more connection, more heart and more juice in the bedroom, shines through her every word. I find her style of teaching to be both deeply transformative and refreshingly simple."

Kim Keller, Certified Tantric Educator and Jade Egg Workshop Facilitator http://kimrosekeller.com/

"Dr. Jane Guyn offers a realistic and often humorous approach in her step- by-step guide to sex planning, making her book perfect for goal- oriented planners. Her easy-to- use exercises, worksheets and affirmations inspire readers to release sexual shame and discover their bliss."

Janet Morrison, PhD, RN, Certified Clinical Sexologist and Sex and Relationship Coach www.janetsexcoaching.com

"With her characteristic love, grace, and gentle understanding, Dr. Jane Guyn guides couples from the blah of a stale bedroom to the luscious joy of reconnecting. Her invitation to create a blueprint for your own bedroom is the hot ticket of your life!"

Dr. Celina Criss, PhD www.delightfulmischief.com/

"Sexless relationships take a heavy toll on people - this is one of the most common clinical complaints that we see in private practice. In Dr. Jane Guyn's book, Too Busy to Get Busy, we find a powerful resource, presented with deep, compassionate understanding, that will change lives."

Sarah Martin, Certified Sex Coach www.goodsexlifestyle.com

"Tired of loving your partner but feeling worried about the sex part just not being there anymore, the way it used to be? I've had great success working with Dr. Jane Guyn's Bedroom Blueprint and its techniques for bringing couples closer. Too Busy to Get Busy promises a safe way to get started back on the road to each other.

Tracy Bryce Farmer LCSW PC, Therapist, Portland, OR

"What a rare and precious treat to get PRACTICAL bedroom advice from a Ph.D. sexologist and sex coach, who is as approachable as your BFF! Spontaneity in the bedroom is wonderful, but it's great to have a plan that suits you. Dr. Jane Guyn's seminal book is your go-to resource for putting the sex and sizzle back into your relationship."

Dr. Claude Cruz PhD author of "Loving Softly" Kindle e-book, Amazon ASIN#B01C12HQS8

This book is dedicated to my beloved Jim,
who has shared the magic of the bedroom with me for over 30 years.

Acknowledgements

I would first like to thank my friends and mentors Dr. Patti Britton and Dr. Robert Dunlap, founders of the internationally praised SexCoachU. The extensive education in the field of sexology that you gave me eventually led me to take on this challenging project. I would never have developed BEDROOM as a model had I not been first educated in Dr. Patti Britton's comprehensive MEBES Model. Dr. Patti, thank you for your inspiration as a professional and as a woman. I am also deeply indebted to my friends at the Institute for the Advanced Study of Human Sexuality, specifically Dr. Janet Hastings Morrison and Dr. Celina Muller. Without your support on a daily basis, my doctoral research and dissertation, which is the inspiration for this book, would not have been completed. Mark LeBlanc, thank you for your support when I first floated the idea of "writing a book about sex" years ago during a business coaching session. You enthusiasm encouraged me. Lou Paget, thank you for your encouragement, support and inspiration. And to my dear friend Jill Smowlowe, thank you for showing me what great writing really looks like.

Table of Contents

Foreword by Lou Paget

If you picked up this book chances are you are looking for solutions, answers, and real people ideas that will give you the personal ability to create and recreate a future bedroom life that works for you and (if you have one) your partner or future partner as well.

Congratulations!!! The first big step to changing anything starts with taking personal responsibility. Not always the most comfy place to be, yet Dr. Jane uses an I'm-in- it-with- you older sister tone through each subject and concept. She strips away the shaming and judgment around our sexuality and focuses on you discovering, knowing, and feeling what is right for you.

Trust me, as one of the best selling authors worldwide in the arena of sexuality, an international speaker and an AASECT Certified Sex Educator, I read and talk about sex information every day. Some really good, some really bad, some so-so. My seasoned eyes can tell you that The Bedroom Blueprint's Step-by-Step format Dr. Jane has created for you is a fresh, unique, and PRACTICAL way to address and revitalize all things connected to you, your sex life, and your relationships.

You have the opportunity to look at where you are now and where you want to be. All guided by a positive, pro-active approach--enough of the rearview mirror method. FYI - The Sex Vocabulary Exercise in Chapter 11 is terrific.

Even better, she speaks from having been where you may well be. Jane lost her connection to and identification of her sexual self, something she had in spades at the beginning of her relationship with Jim. In this book she shares the tools and techniques she used and that her clients use as they journeyed back to fuller, richer, more satisfying sexual connection with themselves and their partners. Luckily for you, you can just read what works and get the benefits of her nursing career's assessment skills, her scholarly work to become a Professional Sex Coach, and her Ph.D. dissertation.

Believe me, it is no small task to make sexuality information and instruction user-friendly, non-judgmental and easy to understand. Dr. Jane puts your hands on the steering wheel and your foot on the gas pedal and you can go as quickly as you like or park at any point. This is your journey at your pace.

No matter when or why you are wanting to change things in your life, the answer is invariably in the mirror. Consider this book another mirror that can help you and teach you to create and recreate the connection, satisfaction, and sexual soul that is your birthright.

L. Lou Paget
CEO/President Frankly Speaking Inc.
Chair, National Leadership Council
Program In Human Sexuality
U of Minnesota Medical School
AASECT Certified Sex Educator
International Bestselling Author
www.loupaget.com

Introduction
I'll Have What She's Having

> "One of the most wonderful and terrifying things about life is that we have no idea how it is going to turn out."
>
> Pam Slim, *Body of Work*

It was a typical rainy day in Portland, Oregon and I was shopping for drapes with my husband Jim at Pottery Barn on NW 23rd Ave. I was more a Home Depot/IKEA kind of home decor shopper, but we'd decided to go upscale for this special purchase and I was very impressed with the Pottery Barn customer service we received that day.

We were looking for something light and airy that would also provide a warm, cozy feeling in our room, so that when we spent time there together during the afternoons, I would feel more open and comfortable making love.

As we looked at all the great options available to us that day, a young sales woman came over to help. "May I help you?" she said. "Yes", I said. "We're looking for drapes." She asked what types of drapes we were interested in; would we like something to block the light, would we like linen, would we like something with a simple pattern? I said that the primary purpose of the drapes was to provide a cozy, sexy environment for us when we were together getting busy during the afternoon.

"Of course" said the well-trained sales woman, "That makes perfect sense."

I could tell by her expression that my mention of our sexuality was unusual to her and felt odd. Maybe she would have felt differently had we been a young, hot, obviously lusty couple. But we are "older than God" as our kids like to say and are neither young, hot, nor obviously lusty.

We went about the process of buying the drapes and eventually chose 2 sets in beautiful white linen plus rods, clips, and all the needed hardware. Jim sat down in a leather chair nearby, waiting for me to finish the transaction. He looked at me and smiled and I waved a little bit across the room.

The young sales woman stopped what she was doing with our transaction and looked at me, pausing with her pen in mid-air. Then, somewhat quietly, she said, "Okay, tell me the secret." When she spoke, her voice was different from her "Welcome to Pottery Barn, how can I help you" voice. This voice was real and hushed and sounded maybe a little bit sad. I looked at her and asked, "What do you mean?" And she said, "What's the secret of your relationship? I've never seen a couple like you in all the years I've worked here."

"Well," I said, "Actually, since you asked, I've got to admit that it's sex. We prioritize our intimate relationship as a couple. We're very intentional about it. That's why we're here buying drapes. My husband knows that I like a certain type of environment when we make love. And we decided that our bedroom is too bright and chilly during the day for me to feel really comfortable. We share time together when the kids are gone and we have the house to ourselves.

She said "I get it." (But I think she was a little taken aback. Here's this obviously much older woman talking about sex in

Pottery Barn. Not your typical day at work.) And I told her "The most important thing is really understanding ourselves and sharing that truth with each other - not having sex out of a sense of duty or obligation."

She said that she was still looking for the right person in her life. But she wanted what she saw in us. She wanted to wave at her partner from across the room at Pottery Barn with a sense of knowing. She wanted to feel welcomed. She wanted to be understood. She longed to feel passionate, loved and adored. She wanted a juicy, hot, erotic, supportive, fluid, spontaneous, adventurous and fun-filled relationship.

And it makes perfect sense that she wants this. It's her birthright. It's what she deserves. And, really it's what we all want. But somehow, for most of us, an authentic, satisfying sexual relationship seems impossible to create.

What I didn't tell her standing there at the checkout counter in Pottery Barn was that we'd been through some very dark times (and some very hot times) on the way to this moment of authentic sharing and connection. What she really needed to know was that when things became challenging for us along the way, prioritizing authentic sex and creating a bedroom blueprint for intimacy had really saved our relationship.

A Blueprint for Your Bedroom

When I talk about a blueprint, people know what I mean. A blueprint helps you know how to lay the foundation for your most important projects - the homes you live in, the successes you depend on in all areas of your life and work. But when it comes to sex, you probably never really plan. And I don't mean just plans about pregnancy or STI's. I mean, plans on how you are going to show up, to please and be pleased by your partner. How to embody yourself in a way that transforms sex from something that makes you feel guilty and inadequate to something that leaves you laughing, smiling and melting into your partner's arms.

Planning for sex seems vastly inferior to the passion of the sex you see in blockbuster movies like *The Notebook*. It's fantastic to watch the two main characters Noah and Allie devour each other as he carries her up the stairs in her rain soaked clothes.

I agree that Hollywood sex is fantastic. And it's true that sex in real life is a lot more complicated than it looks on that big screen. But that doesn't mean that it has to fall off the radar completely. Sadly, for many people, for many good reasons, that's exactly what happens. Sex just disappears in the middle of "Too Busy". Usually once it's gone, it's hard to remember exactly why. Was it pressure from work? The stress of parenting? Feeling hurt when your partner made a comment about someone else's body? For many people it's hard to remember the last time sex was great or even good.

So, how about you? How's your sex life? If your answer is somewhere between awkward, non-existent and soul crushing, you're like many of the people I see as a Professional Sex Coach in my downtown Portland Oregon office.

There are lots of reasons you might be struggling with this incredibly common (and seemingly impossible to solve) problem. It could be because:

1. **You feel out of shape and unattractive.** You don't like seeing yourself naked during sex (or even in the bathtub.) In fact,

you don't want your partner to ever see you with your clothes off. Or, you feel that your partner isn't attracted to you anymore or that your partner finds other people more attractive than you are. This makes you feel terrible.

2. **You're entering menopause** and your body is changing. You're thick around the middle, which makes you feel unattractive. Your libido (a fond friend since your teens) has vanished - seemingly into thin air. You don't feel aroused anymore no matter how you try to conjure a fantasy. Hot flashes have started to keep you up at night and you feel too tired, irritable and turned off for sex. You're wondering if this is your new "normal". Or, your partner is struggling with menopause and you don't know how to handle it.

3. **You're a guy going through "andropause"** - a decrease in your hormonal levels related to aging and you feel a loss of virility and empowerment. You feel insecure and embarrassed but you've never heard anyone talk about these kinds of changes in the media or in your circle of friends.

4. **You are exhausted** from your busy, demanding job and the emails, project deadlines and virtual meetings you're managing. Maybe things have become so overwhelming that you can't keep your eyes open when your head finally hits the pillow. You don't even have the available bandwidth for a quickie.

5. **Your erections are unreliable.** Maybe you've talked with your doctor about the problem but the meds are expensive and sometimes they don't even work for you. You've gotten uncomfortable side effects from the meds in the past and

they're incredibly expensive at your local pharmacy. It seems like a waste of money. But, you're worried that your partner is going to get fed up and leave one of these days if you don't perform better in the bedroom. The whole thing makes you feel bad. It's started affecting other parts of your relationship. In fact, sometimes you pick a fight in the evening just to get sex off the table. This leaves you feeling isolated and alone. It's a whole lot easier (and less embarrassing) to watch something on Netflix than it is to talk about the problem.

6.   **You have a lack of privacy** in your home. Every time you go into your room does someone come barging in? There's no door lock. Or if there is a door lock, someone is always pounding at the door when you go inside. Maybe your home is cluttered and unorganized and you don't feel sexy there at all. When you go into another environment like a hotel room all of the sudden you find your sense of sexuality again, but in the environment where you live, you're completely shut down.

7.   **You just had a baby** (or even twins!) and you're overwhelmed with all the energy it takes to get through each and every day. Maybe you never get a minute to yourself because your baby, or toddler, or little child is always climbing up into your lap and sex is the last thing on your mind. You're juggling responsibilities at work and at home or you're feeling the isolation of one day after another alone taking care of the kids.

8.   **Infidelity has rocked your world.** Perhaps the worst of it is over and you're both committed to your relationship. You're even seeing a really great counselor now. But somehow the counselor never talks about sex. She helps you talk about things that happened when you both were much younger,

which is really helpful in understanding why you do stuff. You know that's important, but right now you're just trying to figure out how to take your clothes off together. You feel incredibly confused. You miss the way you felt before everything went down. Will it ever be good or is this thing over?

9. **You've been struggling with a chronic disease.** Maybe something like diabetes, lupus, chronic fatigue, fibromyalgia or even the after effects of cancer treatment have derailed your sexual connection just when you need it most. Why didn't your doctor tell you about the sexual side effects of your medical problems? At least then you would have known what to expect. You want to stay connected with your partner, but the exhaustion and pain make it almost unbearable.

10. **You are dealing with grief.** Maybe you're grieving the loss of someone very close to you. You crave touch, love and connection but your sexual energy is buried beneath the sadness. Your partner supported you in your grief for a while, but lately you've been getting a lot of pressure to get over it already. This just makes you feel distant and more alone. It definitely doesn't open you up to sex.

11. **Depression is a constant companion.** Or you're feeling down all the time even without a reason that makes sense. Your depression is affecting everything – parenting, work, keeping up with the house and the bills. You've heard that sex can help improve mood and decrease stress but getting there is an absolute impossibility.

12. **Sexual assault has been a big part of your story.** Maybe right when you let yourself go with your partner you think of

what someone did to you in the past (so wrongly, so horribly). Things that seem so easy to others trigger terrible memories and you can't figure out a way to tell your partner what's happening in your head and in your heart. It almost feels like the abuse still lives inside your body. Sometimes you try to make it better by talking but your partner gets hurt or offended when you say something and you feel like you need to keep it in, shutting down your sexual connection today. There's nothing you can do to change the past but how can you get it out of the present?

13. **It has been literally years since you felt sexually attracted to your partner.** You love each other but the sex part stopped happening a very long time ago. You worry that you're going to lose your relationship for something that doesn't even matter to you at all. Why does your partner focus so much on the one thing you can't give? You do everything else to make things great between you. Is sex so important?

No matter what your sex life is like today, you can create a beautiful relationship that is just right for you in the bedroom. This is your guide to creating a workable plan for a wonderful sex life. If you think that the words "workable plan" and "wonderful sex life" don't seem to go together, keep an open mind. Many of the skills and abilities that you use in the other parts of your life will help you in the bedroom. Lots of people find this counterintuitive, but hang on - it will take shape soon.

As an added benefit to doing this work, you'll release shame in other parts of your life too. In the end, you'll have a whole life that works more smoothly and a sex plan that looks, feels and tastes exactly the way YOU want it to; a BEDROOM

Blueprint™ with your name on it. When you do this work, you'll be ready to step into the kind of life that you authentically desire on the deepest level.

No Magic Bullet

There is no magic bullet. You'll need to put in the time and energy. Creating an amazing sex life is simple (and even logical) but that doesn't mean it's easy. When it comes to sex, we put all sorts of roadblocks up in front of ourselves. If you're like most of us, you know exactly what I'm talking about.

Once you get your BEDROOM Blueprint™ in place you'll be well on your way to the sex life of your dreams, but you won't be finished with your important journey. You'll need to keep looking at your bedroom life to figure out how to grow your authentic connection with your partner day after day and year after year.

For some things in the bedroom, just calling out what's in your way is enough to dissolve barriers. In fact, you'll find that when the shame starts lifting (and it is lessening now) you'll see the walls start to come down.

But for other stuff, you'll need more information, help and support to create what you really want. I need your promise that you won't give up on yourself here. You've got to stick with it if you want the real promise of authentic, yummy pleasure, intimacy and love in your life.

Just the Beginning

Just to be clear, this book is in no way intended to be an exhaustive resource of all things sexual. There is an extensive list of fantastic resources written by absolute luminaries in the field of sexology included for you here in the resource section.

The list is there to help you deepen your very important and very adult education. I hope you read every single book on the list from cover to cover. Even if you don't have time to read them all right now, at least you'll know where to get more information when you get stuck on something you don't understand. Deal?

An Invitation Instead of an Encyclopedia

Instead of serving as an encyclopedia of sex, this book is an invitation for you. You're invited to use the same skills in your bedroom life that you use in the rest of your life. You're invited to jump into this project with the same grounded energy you use at work or at home when you're planning your home improvements, parenting your kids, or planning your Disney vacation. An invitation to plan = good. Yes, it is. Because when you apply those skills calmly and with self-acceptance, you'll heal the parts of yourself that somehow never felt good enough. Those sad, hurt parts of Y-O-U will feel heard, accepted, and included. This is transformative.

I'm here to help you release the shame that you feel about sex so that you can open yourself and declare what you really want; so that you can make decisions about sex as a whole person. Bring down drama and increase pleasure. Make a plan.

How to Use this Book

Too Busy to Get Busy is made up of 14 Chapters that show you the importance of communicating and planning about sex. You will learn about the seven key areas of sex – body, environment, desire, relationship, openness, orgasm and mindfulness. You will create your very own BEDROOM Blueprint™ using that information. And you will create transformation in your life by applying your newfound knowledge every day.

Your Sex Plan – a Project in Three Parts

The book is split into three parts that are set up like this:

Part One: Envision Your Park Bench Moment talks about how sex affects us as individuals and couples now and in the future.

Too Busy to Get Busy Chapter One: Get Real About It exposes how we've been lied to about sex by the media, Hollywood, and our upbringing.

Too Busy to Get Busy Chapter Two: Understand What's at Stake includes the heartbreaking voices of real people living in sexless relationships and discusses the impact of sexual problems on relationship satisfaction.

Too Busy to Get Busy Chapter Three: 'The Talk' Made Easy is about the impact of sexual shame and how critical it is to your happiness to release sexual shame right now so that you can start to get real about sex in your life with a partner or on your own.

Part Two is all about BEDROOM - a new approach to understanding, talking about, and making a sex plan - a BEDROOM Blueprint™.

Too Busy to Get Busy Chapter Four: B = Body is all about body image, erections, ejaculation, labia shaming and other juicy topics. Spoiler alert: we're all imperfectly perfect.

Too Busy to Get Busy Chapter Five: E = Environment is about your sex nest, the where and how of doing it - private, public, risky business or all buttoned up.

Too Busy to Get Busy Chapter Six: D = Desire discusses the touchy topic of getting turned on - or not.

Too Busy to Get Busy Chapter Seven: R = Relationship discusses huge questions of who you're with, and how you're with that person (or persons), and how to deal with sex when you're single.

Too Busy to Get Busy Chapter Eight: O = Openness is all about when you want sexual energy in your life and when you don't and how openness is affected by energy, emotion, experience, eroticism and empowerment.

Too Busy to Get Busy Chapter Nine: O = Orgasm dives into your O, pre-orgasmia, the biphasic nature of the male orgasm and multiples.

Too Busy to Get Busy Chapter Ten: M = Mindfulness reminds you that the biggest sex organ is between the ears and talks about doing a chiropractic adjustment on your negative self talk related to all things sex, plus the wonderful influence of meditation on sex and tantra.

Part Three is called Creating Your Bedroom Blueprint™

In this section of the book, you'll take a deep dive into your unique sexual style and create a full understanding of where you are today as a sexual being.

Too Busy to Get Busy Chapter Eleven: Your BEDROOM Blueprint Guide™ includes exercises and worksheets so that you can see yourself as you really are in this important area of your life. This step-by-step BEDROOM Blueprint™ Guide will help you create your plan. You'll also find a fantastic list of resources that you can use to dig deeper into each of the 7 BEDROOM areas.

Too Busy to Get Busy Chapter Twelve: Your BEDROOM Affirmations gives you great examples of affirmations you can start using today to get what you really want.

Too Busy to Get Busy Chapter Thirteen: Dave & Susie's BEDROOM Blueprint™ Example includes a BEDROOM Blueprint™ for one specific couple to give you an idea of what "done" might look like for you.

Too Busy to Get Busy Chapter Fourteen: Conclusion talks about moving forward and being empowered.

Let's Get Started

I'm thrilled that you are coming on this journey with me. It's my hope that when you embark upon this path you'll trade in your (almost) sexless relationship for a deliciously intimate, authentic life that feeds your soul.

Too Busy to Get Busy is for men, women and couples who've struggled to make The Sex Thing work in the middle of stressful lives and who are ready to feel comfortable, confident and grounded in the bedroom.

Your willingness to take the first step right now shows that you're open to claiming pleasure, intimacy and love (and releasing sexual shame at the same time).

Take a deep breath. This is the start of something really big.

Part One
Envision Your Park Bench Moment

Part 1 talks about how sex affects us as individuals and couples now and in the future.

"May we do whatever we can to eradicate sexual ignorance in our lifetime. May we create, instead, a world in which sexual responsibility, wisdom and celebration prevail."

Dr. Patti Britton, *The Art of Sex Coaching* 2005

CHAPTER ONE

Get Real About It

"Our ideas about sex are so complicated that we make the activity complicated"

Marty Klein, *Sexual Intelligence*

A Sex Plan?

Most of us understand the importance of making a plan. We plan for the summer, look ahead to the holidays or an upcoming launch at work. But for some strange reason, we never think to plan about one of the most important parts of our lives - our sexual relationship. My husband and I were the same way. We liked each other (and sex with each other) a lot. But we lead extremely busy lives. I was a nurse who worked on and off in public health, hospice and case management. Eventually I started a small school fundraising company selling imported piggy banks. He worked in a busy clinic taking great care of a wide range of patients.

Why Not Sex?

At some point along the way I realized that what I was very interested in was human sexuality. Sex is such a fascinating topic. It involves everything we are including our bodies, minds, spirits, hearts and relationships. And yet the topic is taboo. I remember making offhand comments about sex to women friends over the years and getting strange responses.

Once I was sitting by the fire having a glass of red wine at a friend's house when her handsome husband came home from a four-day business trip. Jokingly I said "Well, I better be going, I'm sure you two lovebirds want to be alone". My friend looked at me strangely and told me that I made comments about sex more often than anyone she'd ever met. It wasn't a compliment.

I felt that even though others found sex to be something very private, it was important to all of us – no matter how seldom we talked about it – or did it. I realized that even though it was considered strange for a middle-aged woman to talk about it—that I was truly interested in sex as a topic.

A Real Education

In my own life, sex had played an important role. I wanted to share that interest with others through writing and coaching. I must say that my now almost 90-year-old mother wasn't too happy about the plan. Nonetheless, I embarked on a journey at the premier sex coaching school in the world - SexCoachU.

I learned many things about sex that I had never even thought to ask about. In fact, it's very funny to me now to realize what an expert I thought I was before I started learning the more in-depth information about sex. I studied sex in some of the sexiest places in the world including Amsterdam, Las Vegas, San Francisco and Los Angeles.

After a time, I decided to do a doctorate in human sexuality at the Institute for the Advanced Study of Human Sexuality in

San Francisco, California. There I conducted extensive research and wrote a 200+ page dissertation about the way marriage and family therapists deal with sex. (Hint: not much, but they are open to knowing more). The content in this book reflects that exhaustive research.

I haven't always been a sexual health coach with a PhD in Human Sexuality, working with couples and training therapists so that they feel comfortable talking about sex. In fact, for many years, I was a stay-at-home mom who cared more about making awesome Halloween costumes for my 6 kids than I did about sex. I spent my time and energy taking care of my kids--fussing over them, thinking about them, planning for them, and reading about their development.

In contrast, I never spent much time worrying about, thinking about or reading about my relationship (and certainly not any time worrying about, thinking about or reading about sex). I pretty much took my relationship and my sex life for granted. We had a hot, sexy marriage. Didn't we?

Hot and Heavy

Our relationship was steamy from the start. When we first met, he was an intern in blue scrubs, clogs and a full beard while I was a student nurse in a snug fitting white uniform, with properly polished shoes and a starched cap that I pinned into my permed hair. He called my curls "crushable" and I melted.

We shared illicit passion straight out of General Hospital - touching each other at any opportunity. Once we even snuck up to the second floor conference room, where he carefully removed my tights and pulled up my dress. There in the dark, we held our breath as the night custodian clattered along with his cart in an adjacent hallway rattling the doorknob before he moved along.

Over 30 years later, I still have the note he wrote me that night hidden in my wallet.

Chemistry Lesson

Our sexual chemistry was a strong part of how we saw each other in those early times. We were drawn to each other with a magnetic pull, an experience that persisted for years. Our love affair continued from a distance through other relationships as we wrote letters and saw each other only occasionally (and without sex). But that passionate gut-check desire was still there.

Married Life

One summer we moved in together and decided by fall to get married, a decision that must have made our friends and family wonder about our sanity.

Married life was a complete change for us. We'd never had a traditional dating relationship; we were lovers first and foremost, two passionate people with a desire for each other that heated up a room. Settling down seemed out of character. But we fell into a wonderful rhythm of passion, connection and communication that deepened our love and satisfaction for many years.

The Cost of a Busy Family

So how did I go from that obsessively erotic young woman to a middle aged housewife who often fell into bed thinking of nothing sexier than the Thin Mint cookie delivery schedule for Tuesday? What moved me to find books about the developmental stages of a toddler or the prepubertal growth patterns of a tween more fascinating than my incredibly handsome husband? What shifted me from longing for nothing more than to be touched, fondled and entered by my Beloved, to wanting only to be left in peace, saying things like:

> "Could we just cuddle tonight?"
> "I mean it, I've got so much going on tomorrow."
> "Not now, baby."
> "Are you trying to make me feel guilty?"
> "Sorry, but I'm really too tired."
> "I love you. Really. I do."

And I did. But I was having a lot of challenges staying connected to myself as a sexual being.

In many ways, I think I just lost track of my true self during my intense mothering experience. Even though we both adored being parents to our 6 kids born over 13 years (three of them adopted), it was definitely challenging. I was submerged in mothering. My identity as Super Mom became so strong over the years that I was very disconnected from myself sexually.

Such a Mom

I felt like such a mom most of the time that feeling like anything else was very tough. Occasionally we'd go to a downtown hotel and remember the "us" that existed in the early days. I remember those weekends. It felt like I was coming out of a fog. By breakfast in the hotel the next morning, I'd shake my head realizing that I'd been a woman and not just a mom. Yes, yes. I remember this.

It wasn't long before I dove back into full throttle mothering when we got home. This isn't to say that moms can't make a great plan to stay connected sexually. But for me, that plan never really materialized during those days.

Things Changed

By all accounts we had a loving, communicative relationship. But as things got busier and busier, things changed. He'd call me from work and the conversations that for years or even decades had been deliciously inviting became more like tactical briefings than sexy chats. When I answered the phone (if I could find it) I was in a hurry, irritated and fraught. Our conversations were tight. No sugar or sweet on my end, or really on his end either.

Hey Baby?

A typical midday conversation between us went something like this:

Me? Well, I'm just cleaning up Cheerios again.
Hey, yeah I'm ok.
Yup, No.
No, I don't need anything at the store.
Fine. Yes, the kids are fine. They all remembered their backpacks today.
Yeah, see you later. Ok.
Bye.

Click.

Sound warm, welcoming and erotic? Nope. Not so much.

After he got home from work, things got better. We made dinner together. He was helpful with the kids. We talked on the couch at the end of the day. We made love fairly often and it was fine.

Stay-at-home Stress Syndrome

But there was something missing. My lack of self-esteem was tough on me. Not that I didn't adore my kids. I totally did. But the stay-at-home-mom thing was challenging. I tried to keep my mind occupied. I read every book under the sun about being a good mom. I worked super hard to make a difference.

After a while, I got a paying full-time job. And we had a nanny, then daycare and all the stresses faced by every other hard working couple with kids.

But by then I was already pretty disconnected from my feminine energy, my sensuality and my erotic voice. And new stressors had taken over from the deliverables of housework and diapers.

A Rude Awakening

As life would have it, there's always someone with sugar in the world. There came a day when I realized that a beautiful co-worker desired my husband. She was the sweet to my bitter. He softened to her welcoming energy.

Despite the fact that I was often distracted and dismissive, I became completely unhinged when I figured out that they'd been talking on the phone and that he'd even kissed her at work before she moved on to her new job.

How had this happened? How had our hot, steamy relationship deteriorated to a place where I could think of nothing to talk to him about but Cheerios while another woman purred into his cell phone?

Stuff Happens

Well, this stuff happens.

It's incredibly common and it happened to us.

Maybe it's happened to you, too.

We had a lot going for us as a couple. We had always been madly in love. We talked every day. We were polite to each other. We were having sex. But, what we didn't have at that time (and we do now) was an intentional commitment to prioritize our intimate connection in a way that worked for both of us in the middle of "Too Busy".

We didn't know how to bridge the gap between the eroticism of our past and this new life where the house was filled with school papers and Girl Scout badges waiting to be sewn onto vests; where I was entering menopause and he was in the middle of mid-life. We didn't have a BEDROOM Blueprint™ to guide us as we navigated our "Too Busy" lives.

Why Us?

As Esther Perel writes in her ground-breaking book, *Mating in Captivity*, "It's hard to feel attracted to someone who has lost her autonomy". Maybe that was it. Or maybe it's just tough to resist the attentions of a woman who sweetly offers to help you get out of the office early so that you can go home to your (irritable) wife.

He says that he never stopped being attracted to me even as they flirted (and I hope that's true), but whatever happened, the truth is that at home we had let true passion get lost between parent teacher conferences and last minute trips to Target to pick up poster board for the science project.

It's fun to laugh at sexy jokes and feel attractive again. Maybe it seems harmless to have fun at work by joking around. You can't blame a guy for wanting to feel alive. Can you?

A New View

Fortunately, we were smart enough to get quality professional counseling and this helped us understand things from our pasts that mattered today. We talked, cried and sought to understand each other more deeply. It was lucky that he and his co-worker never had sex (at least that's what he says and I believed him), but no matter what actually happened, their connection was plenty devastating the way it stood.

We recommitted to creating a fantastic love affair together. We created a deep and lasting understanding of ourselves and each other in all areas of life – not just in the bedroom. As it turns out, I'm happy to say that our moment of truth as a couple actually made us stronger, happier and more resilient.

What I Want for You

We all get lost sometimes. You may feel disconnected from yourself or from your partner. You may sense that someone at work is taking particular notice and it feels good to be seen. You may wonder if you've made the right decision getting married. You may know that you should have "The Talk" about sex but don't know where to start.

This work is for people today who feel the way we did then; people who are losing track of their real wisdom in their relationship, where sexual connection has become a chore, the very last thing on a long TO DO List or not on the list at all anymore.

Pam Slim was right when she said, "One of the most wonderful, and terrifying, things about life is that we have no idea how it is going to turn out."

That's true. You can't see the future.

But one thing you can see is that your relationship isn't going to get better all by itself. Create a BEDROOM Blueprint™, and you'll find yourselves on the park bench of your dreams – two darling little old people holding hands, watching life go by, remembering the beauty, heat and passion of a life well lived and well loved.

Chapter Two

Understand What's at Stake

When sex isn't working, it hurts.

It is estimated that at least 25% of all relationships (married or single) are technically sexless. This means that at least one out of every four couples has less than 6 shared sexual experiences during a year.

Recently I ran across the Reddit.com sub-thread called Dead Bedrooms. Reddit is an anonymous online bulletin board site where people discuss everything under the sun (and lots of things that never see the light of day.) When I first logged on to the board, there were 29,345 subscribers to that particular Dead Bedrooms sub-thread.

A Survey for the Sexless

After reading a lot of their comments, I decided to create an anonymous survey so that I could understand more of what the people on Dead Bedrooms were experiencing. Respondents to the survey gave me permission to use their comments. Below are their unfiltered voices.

The Question: "What does it feel like to live in a sexless relationship?"

Voices from Sexless Relationships

1. That is all I think about.

2. Feeling like I'm carrying around this huge burden/secret.

3. Not feeling wanted.

4. Leaving the woman that I love.

5. Feeling undesirable, feeling like your partner is wasting your life.

6. Feeling your heart ripped out daily by the person you love...... over.... and over.... and over. Feeling yourself being broken and destroyed by someone who "loves" you.

7. No intimacy. Not feeling good enough.

8. The absence of the intense closeness that sex brings, which helps deal with life in general. If all the good stuff in a relationship is like the classical model of an atom, sex is the nucleus - a cluster of energy keeping the electrons of all the other stuff - conversation, support, shared activities - together. Without it, those electrons fly away and are lost.

9. Rejection.

10. The personal relationship is really bad.

11. It's lacking an aspect of being loved leaving me insecure, unattractive, unloved, no bond between the two of us, undesirable, a sense of disgust on his part touching me or feeling me intimately, unwanted and the feeling of just being a friend.

12. Sometimes relapsing into hopelessness.

13. Being horny.

14. Not feeling desired or wanted.

15. Feeling let down, unwanted and unhappy.

16. There are so many soul crushing aspects. The worst would have to be the adage "feeling lonely even when you're together".

17. The crushing of my self-esteem.

18. Feeling unloved and unattractive, and how destructive that is to your self-worth.

19. Feeling unloved, unwanted.

20. Always feeling unwanted.

21. Rejection and frequent broken promises.

22. I do not feel loved.

23. Isolation, destruction of self-esteem, never feeling complete, helplessness.

24. Feeling of not being desired.

25. That it seems to automatically mean an intimacy-less relationship. We have none. I have a female housemate who I love to bits who walks around the house naked a lot, and we have a kid together.

26. Is knowing that if or when you cheat you are the bad one, it doesn't matter the situation, if you are the male in the relationship.

27. Not being satisfied.

28. The lack of sex that results in resentment and self-loathing.

29. Despair.

30. Your own desire to have sex.

31. The feeling of being trapped. We have children. I'd file tomorrow if we didn't have them. I know that the best thing for me is to leave, but I also know that having both of us as full-time parents is very good for them. (We don't fight or snipe at each other.)

32. She doesn't see anything wrong/doesn't care enough to make any changes.

33. The loneliness and rejection.

34. Thinking about sex all the time.

35. The constant frustration of feeling undesired.

36. Lack of a connection to my partner. She treats it like a chore.

37. It's soul crushing.

The Journey Begins

You're on your way back home to loving sex. I've learned that if you're waiting for that overpowering sense of hot, passionate "strip my panties off me" longing to arrive, you may never have sex again. Don't give up sex in despair and spend your time mourning for the lusty love, youth, connection and aliveness you've lost. This is the way back to eroticism, connection and passion.

It's the path to hot, steamy sex. Yummy deliciousness. You can do this. You can have the best sex of your life. Your journey is just beginning.

By looking deep within yourself and determining who you are in the seven key bedroom areas you will know yourself and express what you need. Really.

Stories from the Bedroom

I share the personal bedroom stories from clients and friends in this book. I am grateful for the permission I was given by these people to use their personal stories. Their names and personal details have been changed to conceal their identities but not to the point of inaccuracy.

Ready to Join the Movement?

It's time for us to start talking about sex (or the lack of it) in our lives. And, it's time to release sexual shame.

This is not about adding sex to our long list of "To Do's". This is not about duty sex.

This is about you cultivating a true connection with your partner based on authentic knowing and true connection on the deepest and most pleasure-filled level.

You deserve this.

CHAPTER THREE

"The Talk" Made Easy

Why is it that every time you turn on the TV or go to a movie, there's another hot couple having passionate sex up against a wall or in a sexy hotel room with perfect lighting and erotic energy that's off the charts?

The way Hollywood and the mainstream media portray sex, it always looks passionate, hot AND completely effortless. We all know that Hollywood is selling fantasy, not reality. (At least not the reality we've got going at our house.) But, it still looks pretty darn good at the multi-plex.

What about sex in real life? Could your sex life get better? How would your life change if you knew how to have soul shaking sex on a regular basis? Would your life be different in a week, a month or a year? How would you feel about getting older if you had an arousing, intimate sexual relationship that left you feeling closer and more understood every time you climbed into bed - instead of distant, alone and not quite good enough?

How would you feel, as you contemplate your life and your relationship, if the whole issue of sex miraculously became simple, relaxing, enjoyable and pleasure-filled?

As a sex coach, I help people to answer these questions for themselves so that they can have nourishing, affirming sexual experiences that give their lives real meaning. I hold space for them as they let go of toxic shame. I listen to them as they dream out loud about what they want in their most intimate times of true connection.

Does it usually look like Hollywood Sex? No, it doesn't. (Well, I'm not actually sure what it looks like because I don't watch my clients have sex. We just talk about it.) But it does look and feel like two real human beings who love and touch and greet each other. We work on creating a practical plan (told you it wasn't Hollywood) so that they can establish a great connection in the bedroom and feel confident and comfortable in their very own skin.

If this sounds like something you need, take heart. You can discover how to feel understood, cared for, alive, and youthful (even if you're older than God like I am). You can learn how to feel connected to your partner physically, emotionally and spiritually. You can learn how to feel appreciated by your partner, how to feel less stress in your life and how to feel more confident, joyful, and content.

The Talk

When things aren't going well, how do you bring it up with your partner without making things even worse? The first thing you need to know is the your bedroom connection is 80% you and 20% your partner. Yup. The 80/20 Rule applies in the bedroom too.

I've had so many situations where one member of the couple wanted to bring up the sex problem, and they did; but they did it really poorly. They didn't know how to talk about it and they offended their partner.

And that was all, there was no more talking about it maybe for years or even decades. When the partner later asked, "Why didn't you tell me this was bothering you so much" the first person said, "Well, I did talk to you about it. I talked to you about it back in 2012, or 2002." This is such a lost opportunity.

Don't blow your chance to talk about improving things in the bedroom. When this initial conversation doesn't go well, it's likely a problem with vocabulary or approach. Get this bit right.

This is the good news and the bad news. It means that while you may feel like your partner is the cause of all your bedroom difficulty, you have a lot to do with whatever's going on too.

Your first step is to take ownership for your experience in the relationship. If you're not in a relationship right now and want to be, you get to take ownership too. "They" didn't do this TO YOU. While it's true that you've been misled by the media, Hollywood and likely your own family, you have the capacity right now to make a huge change in your life.

Do your work to understand yourself in the bedroom. Then, go to your partner in kindness and begin the conversation. Be sure to start The Talk by sharing your sincere desire for closeness and improvement in your connection.

Listen. Take it slowly. Get support.

It's a tall order, I know. But sex is a significant part of your life - even if it doesn't seem like it right now. You'll be amazed at what a difference it makes (to everything in your life) when you get this worked out. Don't worry, we'll take this journey together. I'll be here with you every step of the way.

Part Two
Know Yourself in the
BEDROOM

Part two is all about BEDROOM - a new approach to under-standing sex, talking about sex and making your sex plan - your BEDROOM Blueprint™

"If you're anxious about your sexuality, or you're angry with yourself for feeling (or not feeling) a certain way, or you're ashamed, what you will often do is put that feeling about your sexuality in a box and hide it somewhere deep inside you."

Emily Nagoski PhD, *Come as You Are*

CHAPTER FOUR

B = Body

> *"Your body feels how it feels. Sometimes it gets excited Sometimes it doesn't. Do you trust its judgment?"*
>
> Marty Klein PhD, *Sexual Intelligence*

When many people think about sex, they only think about the body. Sure, the body is where sex happens physically, but people just assume it starts and ends there. Throughout this book, I'm going to encourage you to expand your thinking about sex beyond the body to six other equally important areas. Sex really is multifaceted, and it includes our whole experience as human beings. Still, there are many barriers to sexual pleasure and the BODY, so let's talk about it.

Don't just say it

Before you go any further, we've got to discuss the words you use when you talk about your body - your sex vocabulary; that's what you say when you're describing your sexual anatomy and sexual activities. If you "just say it" you may deeply offend your partner without even knowing it. If you never say anything you run into the same miscommunication problem.

Why do words matter when it comes to talking about sex? Well, most of us learned words about sex and sexual anatomy when we were young teens and pre-teens. This coincided with the time when we were becoming aware of our developing sexuality. Our lives were packed with emotion and embarrassment. We may have been traumatized or bullied on the middle school bus. Sexual shaming may have been part of our lives – it's rampant during this time of life for lots of people. And if you're like many of us, sexually specific vocabulary got filed away under the "inappropriate" or "private" parts of your psyche. When we didn't know a sexually specific word, a neighborhood friend likely filled us in, but the words were never properly aired in our lives.

Fast forward to adulthood. You're in an arousing situation with your partner. You want to touch your partner's genitals and you say "can I stroke your...?"

Hmmm...what word to use? Don't want to sound crass (or like a prude). What words does your partner use? Can't really ask your partner right now because it will ruin the moment. So, you think that you'll remember to talk to your partner about it another time. Of course, that time seldom comes. There's a fantastic but simple exercise in Chapter 11 that will help you clarify a comfortable sex vocabulary.

Don't pass over this exercise. As simple as it is, it can make a huge difference in your sex life. Sometimes people haven't created a shared vocabulary for talking about sex before they become intimate. They end up saying something that makes the partner feel just creepy. And that shuts down the conversation.

Take a look

Now that you've got an agreed upon vocabulary for talking about sex and your sexual body, let's dive in.

It's important to know and understand how your body works. I'm always amazed at how many adults don't really know what their genitals are like on the inside or even on the outside.

Take time to learn about your body parts and the body parts of your partner. A complete review of sexual anatomy is beyond the scope of this book, but we'll go over the body parts that people ask me about most often.

But before we do that, I want you to get in touch with your own body. Take a look. See what you've got. In Chapter 11, as you create your own BEDROOM Blueprint™ you'll get a chance to understand the way you're seeing your body today and how the way you see your body may be affecting the way you show up in the bedroom.

You - up close and personal (an abbreviated lesson)

The Clitoris (no, it's not the Devil's Doorbell)

The clitoris is a wonderful, misunderstood part of a woman's body. While the clitoral head is seen externally on a woman's body, the clitoris actually includes an extensive network of nerve fibers throughout a woman's genitals. For practical purposes, this means that the exquisite pleasure women derive from clitoral stimulation extends beyond the area of the clitoral head.

If you are a woman or you have sex with women, here's another great opportunity to make a plan with your partner. Some women totally love direct clitoral head stimulation. For others, the clitoris is way too sensitive for anything even remotely direct. Learn about your body (or your partner's body). Use the resources available to you here to get more information about how the clitoris looks in 3-D. It's an amazing part of the body that extends into the vaginal roof, the labia and beyond. The take away here is that a woman can learn to experience pleasure from her body that is related to clitoral stimulation and also to touching and stroking other parts of her body - inside the vagina, on the labia and in or around the anus. The neural network that makes up the clitoris is extensive. This is a good thing.

A simple exercise in Chapter 11 will help you get in touch with your genitals in a new way--without shame or embarrassment.

Many women are very shut off from feeling pleasure in the clitoris or in the genitals at all. If this is you or your partner, the first thing to do is to let go of shame about it. Give yourself permission to re-learn pleasure.

The G Spot

We will talk a little bit about the G Spot during the exercise in Chapter 11. The G (or Graefenburg) Spot is an area of spongy tissue in the upper wall of the vagina that is very pleasurable to touch for some but not all women. Sometimes when you touch the G Spot area, a woman may feel like she needs to go to the bathroom.

Female Ejaculation

G Spot stimulation leads us to another very interesting aspect of female sexuality - female ejaculation or "squirting". This release of fluid during sexual stimulation has been in the press a lot lately. Many see this as every woman's birthright. Others see it as a simple release of urine. Recent studies have identified prostate specific antigen in female ejaculate. The fluid comes in part from the woman's Skene's glands which are homologous to the male prostate. This area is also referred to as the female prostate.

Don't let the idea of female ejaculation make you feel bad about your body. If you experience squirting and like it, great! If you don't experience squirting and like that, also great!

Don't put yourself down about what your body does (or doesn't do) right now. You can explore your female fountain by stimulating your G Spot and releasing and relaxing your pelvic floor if you are hoping to learn to squirt.

Remember however that this is not a sex contest. You are wonderful, yummy and delicious just the way you are.

So Many Lubes

There are so many lubes! Which one's the best?

Water based: From liquid to gel, water-based lubricants are lightweight, condom compatible, clean up easily, and can be used safely with sex toys. Not as good for hand jobs, but good for anal play.

Silicone based: Silicone-based lubricants are super slick, extremely long-lasting, made for water play, latex-safe, non-silicone toy compatible and scrub off with soap. Good for manual, anal and vaginal play.

Glycerin based: are not recommended. They have a sugary base and can cause yeast infections in women.

From the Kitchen

Coconut Oil: I like organic coconut oil. It's great for your vaginal chemistry, it's non-toxic and it's food grade. It's even edible! You can use organic coconut oil on your skin after the shower and put a little bit in your vagina at that time to keep it feeling good. Not for use with latex, rubber, or polyisoprene condoms or toys.

Choose a lube and use it liberally. I like it when my clients keep lube right at the bedside during times of intimacy – even when you don't think you are going to need it make sure that you have plenty of lube there. There's nothing like getting worried about getting dry during sex to ruin the fun. And definitely stop the action and add lube if you start to feel too much friction.

Back Door Open?

It's a perfect time to talk about anal sex, since we just finished talking about lube. If anal is on the menu, make sure that you use plenty of lube. It's best if your partner inserts just one finger to help you relax as you start out. Don't rush. Communicate clearly. Take it slowly. Don't assume that because you dug it last time you'll love it again tonight. Listen to your body and to your partner.

Like anything in the bedroom, the key is permission and authentic pleasure. If you don't like anal, you don't ever have to do it.

Oral Sex

Kissing of the genitals is a beautiful, pleasurable way to please a partner. Sometimes a client will ask me if they need to do oral sex until their partner has an orgasm. My answer is a resounding "No!"

When we put "shoulds" on sex the fun goes out of it. Kiss, touch, lick and suck your partner's genitals for as long as you both enjoy it. That's all.

Yummy & Delicious = Clean

Clean up before sex unless your partner specifically suggests that you to go to bed without it (and some people do love that). A quick washcloth job can work wonders for men or women. For the lucky ones with a warm bidet toilet seat cover, enjoy the spray.

Hygiene Matters

For guys this means A SHAVE and a thorough SHOWER. BRUSH YOUR TEETH. Women--stubble on your legs can be a big turn off. Keep your girlie bits beautifully groomed. Mouths, legs, chins, genitals—these things go together beautifully when everybody brings it fresh.

Some people ignore hygiene and then complain about an unreceptive partner. This happens all the time. It's not rocket science. Get this part right.

If your partner comes to bed unwashed and unappealing to you, suggest a bath or shower together. Or get out a soapy washcloth and make cleaning up part of getting ready. Suds are sexy.

Health Matters Too

Overall physical well-being is a huge part of sex. The same things that give us longevity and health; like exercise, yoga, eating right and taking care of our skin improve our sexual experience too. You may want to include a general health goal in your BEDROOM Blueprint™.

Changes after pregnancy and birth affect a sexual relationship as well. For both members of the couple, pregnancy and birth have a huge effect on sex. There are obvious changes in the woman's body during the pregnancy. Following the pregnancy, many women have changes in their abdomen, breasts, genitals, legs and skin. Sometimes these changes impact sensation; often the changes impact self-esteem.

Sometimes their partners are critical after baby arrives. This can have long lasting effects on how she sees her body. If this is your experience, just know that lots of women are very sensitive of any criticism of their body in that post-partum period. Here's another opportunity to add detail to your BEDROOM Blueprint™ at the end of the book. It's very important to talk about how you feel when your body changes.

Menopause and Sex

Many women are not completely aroused before they have intercourse. In fact, in many cases, it's all over before she's even ready. This happens to women of all ages, but the hormonal changes of menopause significantly impact sexual receptivity in women. Menopause causes other not-so-sex-friendly symptoms too - like hot flashes, irritability, difficulty sleeping, irregular bleeding and changes in libido.

Menopause is a very challenging time for some. If you or your partner are going through menopause right now, the best thing for you to do is to focus on your general health habits: eat a great diet, get daily exercise, tend to your beauty needs, have sex and meditate. You're experiencing a lot of change in your body chemistry right now. But, by taking care of yourself overall, you'll get through menopause with more comfort.

Vaginal dryness can be a problem. Dryness is typically the result of a lack of the proper amount of foreplay before intercourse; 20 minutes is the minimum amount of foreplay I recommend.

When I say foreplay, I mean erotic, sensual, non-intercourse touch. When most couples don't spend more than 10 minutes on the entire sexual experience, (more like 7 minutes total on average), I know that most women aren't getting the foreplay they need to have great, juicy sex.

When vaginal dryness shows up use lube without shame. This addresses the issue of vaginal dryness, and increases overall pleasure.

Pain During Sex

I mentioned earlier that some women experience very significant sexual pain. This is common in women after chemotherapy for cancers of various types. Women also experience sexual pain for other reasons.

There are two words used to describe sexual pain in women:

- **Dyspareunia:** which is a general term including any pain with intercourse including vaginal pain but also including deep pelvic or abdominal pain during intercourse, and

- **Vaginismus:** which describes a tightening of the vaginal opening. It gets so tight that nothing can pass through that opening--even something as small as a tampon. Vaginismus can be triggered by deep abdominal pain as a protective mechanism.

I've had clients tell me that sex feels like someone is rubbing shards of glass on the inside of the vagina during intercourse. How incredibly difficult.

Both dyspareunia and vaginismus should be taken seriously. Sex isn't supposed to hurt. Please seek the care of a sex positive medical provider or pelvic floor specialist if you experience pain during sex. For specific information about sexual pain, visit the Mayo Clinic website listed in the resource section at the back of the book.

Some women use estrogen based creams to counteract this problem. However, women who have a history of estrogen sensitive cancers are justifiably concerned about adding hormones of any kind to their bodies. There are effective, non-hormonally based products on the market that are available without a prescription.

Some women swear by the powerful healing effect of Jade Egg work on vaginal health. Jade Egg work is a process by which a smooth egg shaped piece of jade or another stone is gently inserted into the vagina. Wearing the stone is said to improve vaginal ("yoni") health by balancing energy and creating healing. Check out the resources to find out more.

Other women seek the help of Pelvic Floor Physical Therapists to address vaginal pain. Check out the resource area at the back of the book to find out more.

Health Problems

Health problems can impact how you feel about sex. Chronic illnesses like diabetes, lupus, chronic fatigue syndrome, fibromyalgia, and chemotherapy have lots of sexual side-effects. If you are faced with significant health problems, be sure to remember the healing effect of having sex. It may be tough to get interested, but your body will love you for it.

Just for Guys

Body issues around sex aren't just limited to women. In fact, men are known to have a lot of insecurity about their bodies - typically their penis size, shape, length, girth, testicle appearance and erection quality. Women often don't understand how significant this issue is for men.

I have an office in downtown Portland, Oregon; and in my office I have a little table with a dildo on it. The dildo is the size of the average male penis when erect, which is about five inches long. It's not a very big dildo if you compare it to dildos from a sex store. I have it there so that men can see what the average penis size really is and get real.

A Normal Sized Penis

Because if men ever go into a sex store or if they watch pornography on the internet, they're going to see some gigantic penises being displayed; they are just not the normal size of a typical penis.

Many men feel incredibly inadequate about their penises. Even men who have very large penises have concerns about them. This is often because they've had experiences where they were supposed to be the ideal - what women want - but these men have been rejected by women because they are "too big". Self-acceptance is an incredibly important message for men about their bodies.

So, penis size, penis shape; how the testicles hang down or don't hang down - these things are impactful for men. Men also have a lot of concerns about their abdomens, their chests - whether they look buff. The body image issues that women have been struggling with for years are hitting men hard these days.

Hard On Playing Hard to Get?

Erectile problems for men are very common. In fact, for men over the age of 45 there is a likelihood that 50% of those men will have erectile problems to some degree. This is nothing to be ashamed about. Many men have erectile problems at some point during their lives.

For men the quality of their own erections is a very critical aspect of sex. If you're a man and you're not producing an erection when and how you want to, this is devastating.

Aging Manhood

Erectile problems have to do with the aging process; including issues of vascular insufficiency and hormonal concerns. It is important to get your testosterone checked if you're having problems with your erections.

The Blue Pill

There are very well known medications on the market for men with erectile dysfunction - Viagra, Cialis and Levitra.

The medications facilitate your erection but they don't create your erection. The erection is based on arousal and libido. For a man who does not have arousal or libido, these medications aren't effective; but they can still be tried in someone who has a low libido and is struggling with erectile function. This is because sometimes just having that increased blood flow can increase your libido; but they're not a libido medication.

Other Options

Also available for erectile concerns are what's called a **'penis ring' or a 'cock ring'**, This is an elastic type of a ring that goes around the base of the penis, or around the base of the penis and the testicles. It causes the blood to be contained within the genitals. When blood is flowing to the genitals it gets trapped there. This allows you to maintain an erection with proper stimulation.

There is another tool called a **'vacuum pump',** and there are some fantastic ones on the market. They are battery operated and they are not painful at all. The pump is just a cylinder that goes over the penis. There is lubrication on the internal part of the cylinder. It causes an erection using a vacuum process. And then there is a penis ring that goes nicely around the penis, and maintains the penis in an erect condition.

Another option is the **injection of the medication Alprostadil into the penis.** This medication will cause an erection that will last for several hours, even after orgasm and ejaculation for the man.

Sexual Side Effects of Other Meds

Some things as simple as medications can definitely affect erections in men. The **SSRIs** that are commonly used to treat depression and other emotional concerns are one example. They can be very tough on erections and cause erections not to occur, even when the man is adequately stimulated or really desirous of being with a partner. In addition, **blood pressure medications** can decrease erectile responsiveness.

Chronic Diseases

Other things that change erectile response in terms of the body are **chronic diseases such as – diabetes, heart disease**. Illnesses that affect the vascularity of the your body can definitely decrease erectile responsiveness.

Joe was a 42-year-old gay man who came for help because he had trouble getting erections when his partner was there and they were ready to make love. He had erections when he woke up in the morning but during sex, he had trouble getting hard.

They were attracted to each other and they were fit, healthy people. His doctor said that he had no medical reason to lose his erections. Everything checked out fine.

As time passed, and his erections continued to fail him, he felt very intimidated by the idea of becoming naked and disappointing his partner.

His partner was very understanding and really wanted him to feel comfortable. He wasn't trying to pressure him in any way, but he loved sex with him and was hoping they could resolve this issue.

When Joe came to me, he was very concerned. One of the things we talked about was his self-pleasuring (masturbation) practice. He told me that he did not have a self-pleasuring practice at all. He felt it was almost like cheating, so he would never masturbate because he was in a relationship.

Great Homework

One of Joe's early homework assignments after we was for him to develop a masturbation practice. Luckily, his partner was very supportive. He developed his masturbation practice and started working on his erections by himself.

He had good erections when he was self-pleasuring, but when he got into the situation with his partner, he would be intimidated. Sometimes his erections would disappear at the moment of truth.

I suggested he use a cock ring so he could maintain his erection. The cock ring is carefully placed around the penis and the testicles to maintain the erection. This worked really well for him. In fact, his nervousness about his erections disappeared with the cock ring and he and his partner were both very happy with the results.

A hard penis is a relaxed penis

A hard penis is a relaxed penis. What I mean by that is that the body is designed to engorge the penis with blood and create an erection--but not when stress is there. In order for an erection to be produced, you can't feel threatened.

This is completely natural. If you didn't lose your erection during stress, you'd be in trouble if you were having sex and something dangerous interrupted you.

Pleasing His Prostate

The male prostate is a wonderful area of pleasure for many men gay and straight. The only challenge is that the prostate is located inside the anus.

Hmm...no go zone?

Nope! With permission, enter your male partner's well-lubricated anus with your finger and see if he likes it. You're feeling for an area inside that's firm and smooth. It's on the tummy side of his body.

There's no harm in asking. And he might have been hoping you'd give it a try for a long time. If things go well, take your play to the next level with a toy (or a zucchini) and see how he likes that. There are so many fun things to explore!

The Mind-Body Connection

The mind-body connection is part of your sexual response in every way. You can use this to your advantage by taking beautiful care of your body and opening your mind to connection in the bedroom.

CHAPTER FIVE

E = Environment

> *"The quality of women's orgasms is measurably affected by lighting and the "coziness" and beauty of the surroundings in which they are making love."*
>
> Virginia Wolf, *Vagina*

Create Your Sex Nest

Creating a sexy environment at home is a really easy way to improve your sex life. Looking at your environment is one of the easiest and most effective things that you can do for your relationship. Things as simple as getting rid of clutter in your master bedroom, or making sure you clean the bathroom can be huge turn ons.

If you're a guy who wants to have his partner feel sexy, be the one who puts new sheets on the bed, or the one who picks up things in the bedroom without saying anything. Just do it.

Time for Sex

Some couples don't prioritize sex in their schedule, so they go through a busy day and when they get home they're working through the evening. They finally end up in bed together. She's on her kindle, he's checking emails from work; it's 11:15 and they wonder why they don't have sex. Maybe the TV's on at the same time.

When a couple prioritizes sex, that means that they prioritize it starting in the morning. They intentionally look at their schedule and make sure that their daily agenda allows them to wind down with enough time to have sex. Remember, many women need at least 20 minutes of erotic time before they are fully ready for intercourse.

If you don't go to bed until 10:30 or 10:45 PM and you have to be up and getting ready for work at 5:00 AM, you're not going to have enough time.

Morning Glory?

Time of day for sex is another area up for negotiation. When one member of a couple is a morning person and the other is a night owl, what can they do to get things going?

You need to be honest with yourself about what you want. Could you figure out a way to meet at home for lunch and have sex during the day before you're too tired?

How your smartphone is ruining your sex life

Let's say you've finally decided to have sex when all of a sudden somebody gets a text:

Oh, I've got to check that; maybe it's a work text.
Yes, get the text – it might be your manager.
Nope – it was my sister. It's cool
Back to sex.

Having sex - okay.

It's good, good, good.

Oh I'm going to...

Is that your phone? Who's calling you?

Just a sec – I'll get it.

Dang it - it's a telemarketer.

Shoot.

Want to try again?

Ok. One more time.

Another text.

You gotta be kidding!

More?

No.

This kind of thing happens all the time: the interruptions, the online games, the Facebook updates, the video gaming systems. My recommendation is that you keep the electronics out of your bedroom completely. If you need to use your phone for an alarm clock, make sure it's only for an alarm clock. Make it a priority that you're not going to let electronics get in the way of having a great sex life.

Enough Privacy

Couples need privacy, both auditory and visual privacy, to really be able to let go. A lot of people make noise when they have sex. If you're experiencing real pleasure you're going to be moaning; you're going to be talking; you're going to be sharing, and that's great. When you're talking and sharing about what feels good and you're expressing yourself, your partner knows that they're pleasing you. It's really important to be able to do that.

You've got kids in the other room, or your mother-in-law's in town, and so you aren't able to really be noisy with sex; or maybe your bed hits the wall when you have sex. Or something else is making noise, or people are going to see you, because there's a window; you live on a busy street and you've got curtains that aren't quite right.

Focusing on this environmental piece of the auditory and visual privacy is one of the key elements that you can control when you're trying to create a better sex life. That's one of the reasons when you go to a hotel and you have that romantic getaway, you have such great sex, because there's no distraction. It's set up for sex and connection.

Temperature, scents and sound

The temperature of the room, the scents, and the sounds, make a tremendous difference to many couples. If you're in a room that's really cold, and you want your partner on top of you and to have that beautiful vision; yet it's freezing cold in there, that's just not going to happen. You need to make sure that the room is warm, or you're going to set up some kind of a situation where there's a blanket over you both, and then you won't be able to see your partner. Temperature of the room is really important. Make sure that it feels fresh, with a nice scent; something that **you both like.** This is another area of negotiation.

Clean Up

We talked about this in the chapter about BODY but it bears repeating: unless it is a specific part of your partner's BED-ROOM Blueprint™ to go to bed smelly (and some people love that) clean up before sex! For guys this means A SHAVE and a thorough SHOWER. BRUSH YOUR TEETH. Women, same thing. This is Getting Sexy 101 but you'd be surprised how often this simple tip is ignored with negative consequences.

If your partner comes to bed unwashed and unappealing to you, gently move toward the bath or shower together. Hygiene really matters in the bedroom.

Sound Sex

You can do the same thing with sound. Some people like it quiet; other people like certain kinds of music. That's something that you two can talk about so that you create a space that's just absolutely yummy for you. When you get there it's inviting you, makes you feel welcome, makes you feel like it's the place where you want to have this great passionate pleasure experience with your partner.

Light Me Up

Lighting can create a great sense of connection in relationships - or it can be a detractor.

It's a very important piece for many couples. For example, when you're having sex with someone who is aging, your partner may not want overhead bright lighting on when making love. Subtle lighting, something that's maybe candlelight or lighting on a dimmer switch, might feel more comfortable. Of course there are lots of people who love bright, outdoor, daylight for sex and that's something that you should share together.

Love Shack

Specific places bring up erotic thoughts for couples, places such as indoors, outdoors, free, restricted. People have different erotic thoughts in different spaces and some people are very privacy orientated, while other people thrive on the idea of being outside with a risky business kind of sex experience. You can enjoy public sex without too much risk. One fun thing is to go into your garage, close the garage door and get crazy in the car.

Knowing what kinds of environments are exciting for you and your partner is really an important part of setting up a great sex life.

Baby, baby

I recently worked with a couple who had a darling baby. But this was their first baby together and they absolutely loved him. They lived in a cute, trendy neighborhood in a bigger city. The house had multiple floors in it, kind of an open loft-style place with all sorts of cool bannisters and a really sexy round bed at the top.

Wowza

These two were absolutely beautiful. She was one of the most beautiful women I've ever seen in person, and he was a super smart and edgy science kind of guy. They were a gorgeous, active, sexy couple. And they had a precious little baby.

So here they are now; they've worked out a way to be sexually active and have a fun life despite their busy schedules.

But when they had this baby, the baby was tiny and precious and very needy. He was a baby after all and required lots of care. That's the way babies are, of course.

Coitus Interruptus

They would try to be sexual when they weren't too tired and BAM baby would start to cry. Argh. Go get baby. Love baby. Hold baby. Rock baby. It's all good, but not sexy.

As baby got older, **there was no privacy in the house**. Their house, which had been this fantastic, sexy, open-style floor plan, was now really difficult because there weren't walls where their room was, and he heard them. She'd always been an outrageously hot woman but now felt shy and uncomfortable when baby was awake and they were making love. It became a big problem for them to find time and space for sex.

Hey Roomie

Their relationship started to feel less and less sexy and more and more like a roommate zone. Their frequency dropped because the space was off and their energy was off. When they went away and stayed at a hotel they were fantastic; it was sex-on again. But they had trouble maintaining a sexual connection in their own environment.

This couple both worked remotely, with their computers and smartphones in and around the bedroom. Before they were even up it was, "Oh my God, I've got these things happening already. I haven't even had a cup of coffee before I know that I'm behind today."

Rise and Shine

One of the things that we developed as a strategy was for them to buy an actual **good old-fashioned alarm clock**, so that they could wake up in peace.

The other piece was getting a lock on the door so that in the middle of a great, hot, incredibly arousing sex scene, they didn't get interrupted by their toddler saying "What are you doing to Mama?"

Having a place for their sex toys. They had a great sex toy collection, and they didn't want to have their little boy – it'd happened one time – bring their double-headed vibrator out and ask, "Mommy, what is this? What's this thing for?" in front of company, which was both hilarious and horrifying.

Because environment was an issue for them, they used environmental strategies so that they could let go sexually and enhance their love making. They added things like sex pillows or wedges (that don't look so sexual) so that they could enjoy different positions.

There is gorgeous sex furniture that you can buy, but just this one little pillow was a great addition to this couple's relationship. There's a place to find this great bedroom addition in the resource section at the back of the book.

Not Just Candles

Creating a romantic environment for sex isn't just about lighting candles or running bath water. It's the whole way we live. The entire house is really part of it.

Chicks in the Nest

Sex nesting brings to mind how distracting having children can be. Often people complain their sex lives are damaged after they have kids because their focus changes. I think that when you work on the environment, you show your partner that you have a commitment to sex being important.

There's a great exercise in Chapter 11. Don't skip this one. Environmental shifts are some of the easiest BEDROOM Blueprint™ changes you can make.

How Shui is your Feng?

Even getting a Feng Shui person, an organizer, or an interior designer to come in and help you take a look at the space where you're making love can make a big difference.

Stash 'n' Dash?

Many people have prioritized other things over their own sex life. When company's coming over, it's common for people to do the "stash and dash".

"What's the stash and dash", you ask? Well, you dash around your house gathering everything that's out of place and then *stash it into YOUR OWN ROOM*, because you know that your visitors won't be going in there. Your bedroom becomes a repository for the junk in your life.

That's just the absolute worst thing that we can do to our sex lives, is to literally junk up our life with stuff.

Get Rid of Clutter in Your Bedroom

Get the stuff out of your bedroom – if there are newspapers or magazines, clothes that need to be folded, pieces of work that the kids brought home from school, fundraising stuff, or work stuff, all of those things need to be at least out of sight, and even better, out of your room completely. Energetically they can throw off your erotic flow, and it's really key that you keep your erotic energy flowing in all of your life, but certainly in your bedroom.

CHAPTER SIX

D = Desire

> *"Many women describe the loss of sex drive as a loss of part of themselves."*
>
> Laurie Mintz PhD, *Tired Woman's Guide to Passionate Sex*

The Notebook and other Hollywood Fairytales

Have you seen the movie *The Notebook?* Do you remember "that scene"? The beautiful young couple Allie and Noah, (played by Rachel McAdams and Ryan Gosling) see each other in the rain after a long absence. She comes into the door and they just dissolve into consuming passion. They're hungry for each other, clamoring for each other. He picks her up and carries her up two flights of stairs as they kiss, then takes her on the bed, and she's ravenous for him. They strip their clothes off and have this incredibly hot sex. Wow. I want that.

Hot Stuff

Talk about erotic. I use this scene when I train therapists about sex. Sometimes I'll say "Have we seen enough?" as we watch together and they're like, "Nope, nope, let's keep watching." It's very funny, because no one ever tells me to turn that scene off.

It's an incredibly hot scene. Even the gay men in my groups want to watch it. It's great.

We've been taught by the media, Hollywood, and our upbringing that this is the kind of erotic desire that we should expect; that when we don't feel like Allie and Noah something is wrong, and we don't have enough desire to have sex; that desire has to be panting, ravenous, out-of-control, passionate desire from the get-go. The truth is that is just not the reality for the vast majority of couples.

The problem is, when people run into a situation where they don't experience that Allie and Noah level of desire, they have no idea what to do.

Are You Turned On?

So it's like:

"Are you turned on?"
"No. Are you?"
"Yup"
"Okay, I guess we should do it."

Usually one partner is and one partner isn't. The lower desire person is not feeling hot, not feeling aroused, not feeling erotic (at least in this situation) and the higher desire person is there trying to figure out how to initiate sex with somebody who's at the position of stop.

It's tough for the person who wants sex to know what to do. People ask me about desire all the time.

Want More?

How about you? Do you want to want it more?

If so, you're not alone.

We just talked about environment, places where you want to have sex. Like environment, desire can be cultivated intentionally too. Really dig into what turns you both on. Get information from each other about what's arousing to you now and what's been historically arousing to you.

Get Checked Out

Early on, make sure there's nothing medical or physical getting in the way of your arousal. Maybe there's a hormonal difficulty, or a medication with sexual side effects. Maybe it's low testosterone, and your doctor will recommend treatment.

What's the difference between desire and arousal?

You may wonder, how are desire and arousal related? It's an interesting question. You may be aroused by something but not actually desire to have it happen, or you may desire to have something happen (sex with your partner) and not feel physical arousal. Simply put, arousal is more of a physical experience. and desire is more experiential in your heart and head. This doesn't mean that if you're a woman and you're not naturally lubricated that you're not aroused. Sometimes our arousal is a little disjointed. It's ok.

Decide to Want it

Desire is a decision. You decide to allow yourself to be in an erotic situation. You allow yourself get turned on. You have the choice to spend time together with intent to become intimate even if you're not aroused yet.

Sexual Aversion - the short answer

What about aversion? Some people describe having negative physical reactions like nausea or feeling sweaty when they think of being intimate with a partner. If this is you, listen to your body and your heart. Create an intention to release what doesn't serve you.

You may find that you are resisting the intimacy that sexual connection brings. Or, it may be something else. Whatever you do, don't run from your experience. There is tremendous growth available for you here.

Are you reacting to something from the past? When something difficult has happened to you, sexual desire becomes confusing at best and shattering in the extreme. Sexual aversion can result from sexual trauma. Unfortunately, sexual aversion rarely goes away on it's own. In fact, the experts say that it gets worse the more you avoid it. There's a link to an interesting article about this in the resources area. Check it out.

What can you do? Stay in the present. You have a right to pleasure. Don't let the things that have happened to you steal your birthright. As much as your memories may seem real today, what happened in the past is now over.

Find a sex positive professional to support you as you learn more about what this means. Most experts recommend that even if a history of sexual abuse is causing you distress, you will be able to heal yourself by slowly connecting to a supportive partner and replacing negative memories with positive experiences. Keep a record of your responses and share them with a sex positive professional.

All About Gender?

There's said to be a gender difference in arousal and desire between men and women. But there are many, many heterosexual couples where the woman experiences as much or more desire for sex than her male partner. In these relationships, because the culture expects men to be the higher drive partners, the woman often feels shame and embarrassment.

You Started It (or not)

So it's not all about gender. In same sex partnerships, there's often one higher libido partner (HL) and one lower libido partner (LL) too. In my experience working with clients, and in my personal experience talking with friends – one thing holds true. There's a dance of desire and initiation between the HL and the LL partner.

If the couple breaks up, the "lower" can become the "higher" in a new relationship, but in the dance between two people usually one person leads and the other follows in the bedroom. This can be a point of contention. The sexual leader often complains that their partner never gets things going in the bedroom – never initiates.

"Starfishing"

At the extreme, the partner is said to "starfish" - or participate without any engagement at all. This is considered by some to be the ultimate sexual insult. The LL partner may rightly state that "we had sex" but if the HL partner defines the sex as Starfish Sex, it "doesn't count". What the HL partner is seeking (and we all are seeking) is to feel welcomed, celebrated and adored during sex – not just serviced.

Some HL partners even talk about "feeling like a rapist" during sex because the LL partner seems so uninvolved and "just wants to get it over with". The LL partner has said "yes" to sex but is very physically passive and emotionally distant. This experience, while providing physical release, actually leaves the HL partner with a tremendous sense of loneliness, rejection and shame.

Don't Just Think of England

I'm not telling you this to make you feel bad. If you're the LL partner in your relationship, the last thing you want to do is engage in Duty Sex. Queen Victoria is falsely credited with having told uninterested brides to "Close your eyes, open your legs and think of England". Historians dispute the accuracy of that report; the Queen apparently loved sex and had 9 children to prove it. However, the idea of duty sex is still alive and well long after the end of the Victorian Era. Some people still suggest that since your partner "needs" sex, you should "just do it". I heartily disagree.

Blue Balls

In her fabulous book *Come As You Are,* Emily Nagoski vehemently contests the idea that sex is actually a drive like hunger or thirst. She defines it as a motivation. So, your partner may really, really want sex but believe me, your partner will not die without it. If your partner is a male, he will not get "blue balls" and suffer some long term damage to his testicles if you kiss passionately with him and then choose not to have intercourse. Honest.

Theorem of the Blue Balls Debunked

The problem with the Theorem of the Blue Balls, is that it means you've been told not to "start something you won't finish".

Okay, you say. Not a problem. No kissing if you're going to hold me to that standard. No kissing. Also, no touching or hugging because you might "get the wrong idea" and I don't want to go there.

You may have a very motivated partner. You may not be so motivated. You are going to follow my guidance and not just Do It For England. But you want to have a great relationship with a loving Park Bench Moment. What can you do? Here is where we get to the part about choosing arousal.

The real problem with this whole thing is when you enter into this tense sexual truce. You've stopped touching altogether (no yummy French kissing, stroking, light touching, rubbing or holding)–except for heartbreaking Starfish Sex on somebody's birthday or your anniversary.

The French kissing, stroking, light touching, rubbing and holding might get you really in the mood if you did it for long enough. But, since that's off the table, you're left with limited options and no turn on.

Reactive Arousal

This is called reactive arousal. You may want to be connected with your partner, and even intend to have sex, but your arousal happens over time after you've been touching, kissing and stroking for a while. Allowing yourself to experience reactive arousal is the beginning of creating a juicy relationship again. But, you need to make an agreement that just because you are touching, kissing and stroking doesn't mean that you're agreeing to sex.

This agreement will be a part of your BEDROOM Blueprint™. When couples give themselves permission to create arousal like this without assuming it will lead to sex, there's a beautiful increase in intimacy.

Lover's Lookout

Some couples even go places where they know they won't be comfortable having sex to make this a fun game. Drive up to the local make-out place, look out at the view and slowly start kissing, touching and groping each other. Put some sexy music on your phone. Allow yourself to feel pleasure without pressure.

These places are filled with erotic energy. Can you feel it?

High Libido Men and Women

For high libido men and women, desire may be something they fear thinking "Oh I don't want to be turned on right now, but I'm feeling aroused. This is not an appropriate partner for me." Sexuality is powerful and that power feels dangerous sometimes.

Desire Discrepancy

Knowing each other, you can create a plan to nurture compatible desire for you both asking yourself what's been erotic in the past. Check into your lived experience right now looking for your erotic energy. Take time and feel into yourself. See if you can find that energy *in the now* and connect with what's really true for you.

Fantasy

You can use fantasy to stoke your desire. Why not try writing fantasies to help you get in touch with what's inside of yourself erotically? Write about things or people who aren't in the room or circumstances you would never do. Decide if you want to share your fantasies with your partner. You don't have to.

I have a client who gets turned on about confusing stuff. I tell her to welcome her desire. It's just a feeling. She doesn't have to act on it. Ever. And neither do you.

"Hello there, it's your erotic self!"

Desire is just your erotic self speaking up. Your erotic self knows when to be quiet. You've figured out how to stay safe and be appropriate at family gatherings. But when you shut down the whole erotic mechanism inside you, it's tough to access it on cue. It may be messy but saying "yes" to desire when it turns up can be a big "You Betcha" for your love life.

This doesn't mean you have to act on your feelings. When you experience yourself as an erotic person, you grow.

Porn Problems

Pornography is a big problem for some couples. You may feel extremely guilty about watching porn. You may watch porn until you are almost numbed to feelings about your partner.

Traditional porn (Can porn be traditional?) has certain camera angles and sex styles. The sex style is designed to show the action. It's not designed for pleasure.

Maybe porn has caused you and your partner to lose track of what real sex looks, sounds and feels like. When you get into an actual sexual situation you may not even know how to act without porn sex as a guide.

Boner Bummer

If a guy has been watching lots of porn he can even have a problem where he doesn't get erections that are satisfying for him in real life. He may be so turned on by porn that he can't produce an erection with a partner. When it comes to porn, use caution before you proceed. Use porn to arouse you if you want to but your real life is where true connection and intimacy live.

(As a contrast, the Feminist Porn Awards showcase examples of erotic films that go beyond typical mainstream porn. Take a look if you're interested. You may find something that arouses you there.)

Dirty Vanilla

As you begin to explore your sexual fantasies, you'll discover an incredible variety of stimulating possibilities for your life. The trick is to touch in with yourself authentically and share your truth. Things like erotic power exchange (BDSM), threesomes or "moresomes," the sacred sexual practices of Tantra or swinging can fill your fantasies or your calendar.

People don't necessarily want to or need to go to a BDSM dungeon, become part of a tantric sex group or visit a Tantrica or Dakini. You don't need to get involved in wife swapping or polyamory. The only thing to keep in mind is that your sex life needs to fit your own personal values, to be respectful of the needs and values of others and to be safe. With the agreement of your partner, you can create something very colorful.

Maybe this is something that you don't do in real life but you write about in your fantasy journal. Maybe you read erotica to each other about it. You may stay plain vanilla but nobody will know if you're "*dirty*" in your mind - unless you tell them.

What Else Can You Do to Get Turned On?

Great sex is all encompassing. It involves your heart, mind, spirit and imagination. But sex is ultimately a physical act. That's the good news and the bad news. If you're not feeling connected to your body, you'll have challenges. The good news is that diet and exercise are really important to your life in the bedroom.

Eat Your Aphrodisiacs

Eat Superfoods to increase desire and get ready for sex. Create a sexy meal together. It's great for your health, weight and arousal. Plus, cooking is a fun and sexy thing to do. Get cooking and heat up your relationship.

Check out these aphrodisiac foods.

- Blueberries
- Chili peppers
- Almonds
- Pistachios
- Avocado
- Oysters
- Chocolate
- Bananas
- Honey

- Coffee
- Watermelon
- Pine nuts
- Arugula
- Olive oil
- Figs
- Strawberries
- Artichokes
- Chai tea
- Pomegranate
- Cherries
- Pumpkin seeds
- Whipped cream

Pop the Bubbly

Alcohol is relaxing and can help you release your inhibitions, but at its core it's a depressant and actually decreases sexual performance. Use alcohol in moderation for the best sex. But a little bubbly can be a nice touch.

Try Partner Yoga

Partner yoga is a connected approach to yoga that expands the traditional practice of Yoga into the realm of relationship. It's a beautiful practice that will increase your connection with your partner while you open your energy and your body to receive pleasure.

Dance Together

Desire is born on the dance floor. Turn on the music and turn down the lights. If you have privacy, take off your everyday clothes and put on something sexy - or maybe nothing at all.

Use Illegal drugs legally

In the Dead Bedroom survey, participants who were struggling in sexless relationships offered their tips to heat things up. One of the things they recommended was smoking marijuana. With marijuana legal in several states now, you might want to make a trip out West to spice things up. Marijuana isn't guaranteed to turn you on (and it does have some drug effects that you might not like) but it could be fun.

His and Hers

One of the couples I work with is a husband and a wife. The problem with desire in this couple ended up coming to a head after he felt rejected many, many times. He said that every time he wanted to be with her, she was just not at all interested. And she started to feel like he just wanted "it" and not her.

She pulled away from her own erotic edge more and more because it felt like he was putting her down when she wasn't physically turned on.

I explained that it was important for them to realize that she had a different slope of arousal than he did. He could overpower her with his arousal if he came on to her too forcefully. They created a BEDROOM Blueprint™ where he slowed down his advances and she allowed herself to warm up slowly.

Plan It

In this couple's case they made a decision to have a sexual encounter and plan it, not wait and wait and wait for desire to show up. They decided to set up a sex date and a sex space with a nest on the floor including pillows and blankets. Setting up this beautiful nest of pillows and blankets was fun for both of them. They included nice lighting with scents and sounds that were erotic to her – because she's the lower desire person in this relationship. These things really clicked for her.

Outside In

He started touching her on her hands, feet, and head bringing her desire energy from the periphery toward the core with his fingers. By gradually doing this, the lower desire person, in this case a woman, is allowed to energetically connect to a sense of arousal.

When you try to start a lawnmower, sometimes it takes a few pulls on the starter rope. That was the case with this lower desire woman. Once she got going she was great, but it just took time. Don't give up on your lower desire partner if you want to have a full sexual expression.

Many people say they don't have time for sex, but frankly, the studies show that sex only lasts about 10 minutes. For most women, the warm-up time is 20 minutes. So it's over before she's even had a chance to get warmed up. Be patient with the process.

What Other Experts Are Saying About Desire

Rosemary Basson

Rosemary Basson's circular sexual model is different from the way we've thought about sex since the 1960's when Masters and Johnson observed live couples having sex in their lab. The nonlinear Basson Model promotes the idea that your emotional intimacy, sexual stimulation, and relationship satisfaction affects your sexual response in a circular way – the more you open in your environment and relationship, the more aroused you get. This is if you're a woman. If you're a guy, the linear Masters and Johnson model was designed for you. If the Basson model is a good fit for you then emotional intimacy and your relationship satisfaction will increase your sexual arousal.

Esther Perel

Esther Perel takes the opposite approach to your desire. In her book *Mating In Captivity*, she contends that your increased intimacy actually dims erotic tension. She tells you to hold on to mystery within your relationship so that you can cultivate your erotic tension.

Jack Morin

In his book, *The Erotic Mind*, Jack Morin agrees. He says that you experience increased excitement when you're attracted to somebody but can't quite get there. (I'm thinking that's the sexy 20-something bearded guy with the pour over black coffee at Case Study Coffee you see every morning. He's hot but you're 45 and very married. Still exciting. Very.)

Jack Morin's formula tells you that:

Your Excitement = Your Attraction × A Perceived Obstacle.

Emily Naroski

You can look at Emily Naroski's book *Come As You Are* to find out what the scientists are saying about the neuroscience of desire right now. She talks about your Sexual Excitement System (your feelings about that guy at Case Study ie; the gas pedal) and your Sexual Inhibition System (your realization that you're happily married and 45 years old ie., the parking brake).

She says you may have pedal to the metal and your friend may have a harder time getting out of park but that everyone can learn to get going. Naroski tends to agree more with Basson than with Perel or Morin. She says that most women rely heavily on context to get going in the bedroom.

Gina Ogden

Gina Ogden sees desire as coming from a mixture of the physical, mental, energetic and spiritual parts of who you are sexually. She has created a spiritual and metaphysical approach to your desire. She's not so worried about the guy in the coffee shop. She's more about finding a path to your erotic core through a union of every part of yourself and through healing who you've been in the past.

Patti Britton

Patti Britton addresses desire using her **MEBES** model. She encourages you to find desire in the place where your **M**ind, **E**motion, **B**ody, **E**nergy and **S**pirit meet.

For more information about these incredible thinkers and to get the full context of their work, check out the resource list.

CHAPTER SEVEN

R = Relationship

> *"Marriage counselors, labor negotiators, and kindergarten teachers have known it all along: Whenever two or more people get together to accomplish anything, sooner or later there's bound to be a conflict."*
>
> John Gottman PhD, *The Relationship Cure*

Communication in your relationship overall affects sex in many ways. We've talked a lot about negotiation. You can't negotiate if you can't communicate. It's the hottest sex tip I've got: communicate and communicate kindly. Communicate with patience and with consideration to your partner. If you take nothing else away from this book, take that tip today.

Daily Arguments Affect Sex

Couples fight about lots of things: they fight about money, they fight about the kids, they fight about the in-laws, they fight about scheduling, they fight about being late, they fight about clutter, they fight about papers piling up, bills, they fight about who's going to pay the bills. They even fight about vacations.

All this fighting impacts sex. When you decide to have an argument with your partner about something that isn't all that important to you, (and fighting is a **decision** whether you recognize it at the time or not) you've got to remember that you may be making the choice that you don't have sex tonight. Think about that before you pick a fight. I know this isn't always easy. We fight too. But we know it gets in the way of intimacy when it happens.

Sex Fights Are Worse

Fights that have to do with sex are more painful, more impactful, and cause more discord than other fights. Studies show that sex fights cause way more difficulty than other fights in your relationship.

Make Up Sex

Some say that Make Up Sex is a good idea. I think that the damage caused by the fights isn't worth it. Like lots of sex, Make Up Sex really looks best in the movies.

Now, you may have a big fight and great makeup sex afterward. You may say "Oh honey I love you, I'm so sorry" and then have a wildly passionate experience. But the things that you said during the fight are still in your partner's head. And that stuff will still be there the next time you have a conflict and the time after that. You're building a junkyard of bad stuff in there. Eventually, no matter how great the Make Up Sex is it won't do anything to touch the resentment, hurt and loneliness you've created.

Critical Negotiations

If you find yourself fighting dirty all the time, get counseling. Marriage counselors and therapists are great at helping people learn new ways to process stuff. You need to be able to talk with each other so that you can negotiate your lives – including negotiating a sex life that feels good. When couples learn better ways to process daily conflict, they're better at negotiating in the bedroom too.

Negotiation is at the core of all relationships. You negotiate about money, about what you're going to eat, about basic little things. Even things like laundry, shopping, planning next steps on big projects and taking out the recycling come into play. You've got to work together in order to have a great life.

Fight Night

If you find yourself picking at your partner, or being criticized by your partner over every little thing, you're probably on your way to a bad sex relationship and a bad relationship overall. And this is more important in the bedroom than it is in any other part of your life.

For some reason, we think life happens effortlessly without negotiation. Then we're shocked when we have arguments. Insight: lots of couples fight about the little stuff so that the big stuff (like the fact that you haven't had sex in over 18 months) is off the table. No discussion. If you find yourself fighting a lot, ask yourself (and your partner) if your fights have anything to do with sex. Just sayin'.

Oops, I think I'm with the Wrong Person

And then there's the whole issue of the WHO. If you're rocking the single life, are you looking for someone in the future? Who is that someone? How will you know it when you meet the right person?

If you're in a relationship, how are you feeling when you look across the table at that smiling face? Are you comfortable settling into this relationship? Are you feeling committed to this person and making it work?

You may be answering "no" to that question. You might be saying "oh my gosh" I think I've married the wrong person. Sometimes that happens.

If that's the case in your life for whatever reason, I empower you to take care of yourself. Get grounded. Think long and hard. Get support. But if after you've really thought about it, you decide to leave your current relationship, be kind to both yourself and your partner. It's true that your partner deserves to be truly cherished. If you know in your heart that you can never truly cherish this person, it's my opinion that you should let your partner find someone who can.

Why Not Me?

There are significant reasons that you might choose to leave your relationship now.

One is because of sexual orientation. Maybe your sense of who you're sexually attracted to doesn't fit who you're with. You could be a lesbian woman who's married to a man. You might have kids and a whole married life. When you think of coming out and changing your life ("just because of sex") it can feel overwhelming. It's very tough. This is another time when it's helpful to seek the help of a qualified therapist.

Please be kind to yourself. Sex and authentic sexual connection are very important. When you live a life that's misaligned sexually, you damage yourself at a very deep level.

The Affair

Some people leave their relationship because of an affair. Maybe you had an affair, maybe your partner did. Maybe years ago you announced with conviction that if "you ever cheated on me I'd leave you – no questions asked!" Now you are faced with the reality of that situation and are thinking about what to do next.

I helped a couple after she found out that he'd had an affair with a woman he'd met at a convention for work. She found out when she saw a very personal text come up on his phone. They came to me in a state of tremendous upset and dissatisfaction.

Like lots of my client couples, they'd thought about seeking marital counseling, but he felt this was primarily a sexual issue. She was willing to come along to the sex coach in hopes of improving their relationship in this challenging area.

When I first met this young attractive couple, you could've cut the tension with a knife. Into this little office come two people who are attacking each other, not physically, but in every other way - energetically, verbally and emotionally.

Caustic and Hostile

They were caustic and hostile. They put each other down, calling each other names. He was disgusted that she'd only had a few lovers before they got married. He wanted her to be a more willing and adventurous sex partner.

He said that she was great in every other area, but he wanted her to improve in the bedroom. She knew that he'd been upset about their sexual frequency for years. They typically only had sex every 5 – 6 weeks at the most. She'd always intended to make love more often but life got in the way over and over again. For her part, she was furious that he'd gone outside the marriage for sex. She felt betrayed and humiliated. She didn't trust him.

Oh Wow

And I sat there thinking, "Oh wow." The situation was really something else because it was so intense. We went through a process of discussing what they wanted and stepped back from the hostility, anger, and resentment that they both had.

He felt very hurt that she'd never really been open to him as a sexual being. He'd wanted her to have more sex all along and she'd ignored him. In a way, it was like he welcomed the crisis because finally she was listening to him and was there talking to the sex coach.

Take a Deep Breath

Here we are sitting in this room, with the ferns growing and the water flowing and a candle burning, and me thinking "Oh wow, how are we going to get out of this alive?" I asked them to please close their eyes and sink deep into their chairs, allowing their feet to settle into the floor below them, and just to take a deep breath in through their noses, filling their lungs all the way up, all the way up, and then letting it out, very slowly, slowly, slowly, and just to relax into this space, right here, right now. They took three deep breaths together.

I'm Ready

When they were finished, I asked them to please open their eyes when they were ready to be in the room with me and ready to coach with me right now. They opened their eyes, and each of them said separately, "I'm ready."

I asked them then to tell me what their morning would be like if they woke up the next day and a miracle had happened. What would it be like right now in their lives?

She started. She talked about waking up and it was a beautiful morning, the light was streaming in the window, and she had white linens on her bed.

White Sheets

Almost all my women want to have white sheets on their beds. If men only knew this, they'd buy less jewelry and more high thread count sheets.

Anyway, she had these beautiful white sheets, and she woke up, and there he was next to her, and he was just close, and they were relaxed and together, and they were laughing. And maybe they'd made love and they felt close, but there was no tension and no pressure.

His fantasy of the miracle morning was very similar, where they had this sense of being connected and present with one another. They also had a dog they really liked very much, and both of them had the dog in the miracle morning. The dog was in the bed too. And they talked about this fantasy of how they would be waking up just with a sense of beautiful relaxation and connection and no conflict.

It was obvious to me and to them that they both really wanted this relationship to continue. That was very encouraging for all of us, because when they first came in, I thought "Why don't you just skip this office, save the money and go straight to your divorce lawyer? Because this thing's over."

Much Better

Fortunately for them, they were able to see that both had this image and this vision of a beautiful life together, and they continued working on it.

She opened herself to his suggestions about increasing their frequency and trying new things. He learned how to please her. They bought a new sex toy.

They started communicating. After several months, they came into my office laughing, holding hands and looking at each other. Pretty soon, they told me that they felt good and felt complete with our work. As they left my office that day, I knew that their relationship was much better than it had been in a long, long time.

Coloring Outside the Lines

Monogamy isn't for everybody.

I live a monogamous lifestyle but many people don't. Having sex with somebody outside your relationship isn't always cheating. Some of my favorite people make agreements with their partners to have sexually open relationships.

One Size Doesn't Fit All

Sexually non-monogamous relationships are as varied as the people who create them.

You can add variety and ethical intimacy outside your primary relationship if that's what you're seeking. This is called consensual (you have your partner's consent) non-monogamy.

Do you relish the idea of being sexual with other adults – either in the presence of your partner or on your own? Lots of people are creating these unconventional lives today. With good communication skills, you and your partner can create a sexual life together that invites others into intimate experiences with you.

Good Morning!

One of my dear poly friends recently told me that **the difference between polyamory and swinging** is that poly people have breakfast and swingers go home. Sexual expression in polyamory is designed to enhance connected personal relationships while (generally speaking) swinging is primarily sexual and less relational. That doesn't mean that swingers don't make friends with their sex partners and poly people don't have great sex. It's more a matter of emphasis.

A Box with 69 Crayons

That same friend tells me that when she talks about consensual non-monogamy, she thinks of it as having a wonderful box filled with 69 crayons. When she creates her life, she looks at all the crayons in the box—not just the black and white ones the way a monogamous person (like myself) might look at them. She selects the colors with sensitivity to her own needs and to the needs of her partners as she draws a portrait of the possibilities between them. Beautiful.

And?

There are couples who decide that since one member of the couple is **not sexual anymore for medical or other reasons,** the other seeks sexual connection outside the relationship with the knowledge and permission of the primary partner.

When you tip toe (or jump) into a consensual non-monogamous relationship, there are a few things to remember.

1. **You'll need to communicate clearly.** This should happen in all relationships, but those of us in monogamous relationships often skip the communication part (with terrible results). When you venture into consensual non-monogamy, you've got to keep the lines of communication wide open.

2. **Prioritize health and safety.** When you're monogamous, you assume that your partner is too (not always accurate). When you're not, you need to discuss your risk when sharing sexual fluids. Safer sex rules apply here.

3. **Share your expectations openly and with respect**. Again, this is something that everyone should be doing in the bedroom.

4. **Be mindful as you play.** Altering your mental state with alcohol or other drugs in order to loosen up may help you if you're nervous, but you'll be better off in the long run staying clear headed during play at least when you first start out. Call me Mom, but I think this is best practice.

Find more information about creating a consensual non-monogamous relationship in the resource section.

CHAPTER EIGHT

O = Openness

> *"True sexual sharing is an ongoing happening. It radiates throughout your body, your breath, your smile, your smell, your dress, your attitude, your hair follicles, your whole being—in the bedroom and beyond."*
>
> Gina Ogden PhD,
> *The Return of Desire: A Guide to Rediscovering Your Sexual Passion*

What does openness mean when we're talking about sex? I have the wonderful opportunity to be interviewed fairly often on podcasts and radio shows about sex, and sometimes people will ask me about openness.

When people ask me about openness, they wonder if I'm talking about polyamory and swinging. Nope, that's in the chapter we just finished. What openness means in BEDROOM, is being open to your own sexual energy and the sexual energy of your partner.

A lot of my clients come to me with barriers in openness. It may be expressing as a barrier in the body - erectile dysfunction, vaginal dryness or vaginal pain. But when you really dig in, the primary problem is often openness.

When I work with people about openness, we talk about five things:

- Energy
- Emotion
- Experience
- Eroticism
- Empowerment

Energy

Energy influences sex a lot. This includes the obvious lack of energy of an exhausted mom who's caring for her newborn baby as well as the subtle energetic attunement of an intuitive healer in a grove of ancient Coastal Redwood trees or the sacred sexual connection of tantric lovers.

Low Energy

How often is feeling too tired, too busy or too stressed out a problem for sex? For many people, the answer would be the rhetorical "when is it not?" It's a huge problem.

Are you exhausted?

Are you closed down in your energy or just burnt out on a daily basis? Is your level of energy so low that getting into bed and taking off your clothes with the intention of having sex is beyond you?

Our culture supports "Too Busy" as a legitimate lifestyle. But we are not encouraged to make time for sex. When you think of it, our 50% divorce rate isn't that surprising.

Tomorrow Never Comes

When you get too busy you get too tired. It's great to say "This will pass. It's only a couple of years. The job is super demanding and the kids are little. We're building our future here. Later, we'll spend time making love and traveling."

But two years become four and then eight and all of a sudden, you can't remember the last time you had sex. The kids are getting ready to graduate. You have time together at last. You have no idea how to cross the abyss that's grown between you.

Nurture your energy to increase your openness. Take a nap. Get to bed on time. Ask for help. Do it now so that you can make it to your Park Bench Moment. You can be that couple - two darling little people smiling through milky eyes, holding hands with stories of a love affair that lasted forever.

Sexual Energy

The subtle exchange of sexual energy is a beautiful thing. You can find out about practices like tantric sex, Quodoushka and other energetically based sexual practices in the resource section. Some people even learn to have energetic orgasms – orgasms without any physical touching at all. Sexual energy is a powerful aspect of sexual openness.

Emotion

Emotion includes all of the usual players in the bedroom. The emotions that open you up—love, joy and happiness—as well as those that shut you down—jealousy, fear, anger and of course depression.

Difficult emotions such as jealousy or resentment can strongly affect the feeling of being open to sex for a couple.

Mental Health

Mental health concerns of all types have a significant impact on sex. While a comprehensive review of mental health and sex is beyond the scope of this book, when your relationship becomes sexless (or almost sexless) keep mental health concerns in mind. There's a dynamic at play here between sex and mental health—each influences the other.

Get Help

Seek the help of a mental health professional when you sense that mental health issues like depression, anxiety, obsessive compulsive disorder, bipolar disorder or schizophrenia are impacting sex for you or your partner.

Sex is powerful stuff. Mental health concerns show up in the BEDROOM area of openness/emotion. Sometimes mental health issues increase sexual openness to an extreme. Other times they shut it down. This is a place where DIY isn't your best option. Find resources at the back to help you get started.

Everyday Feelings

Emotions influence openness. When I'm angry or jealous or resentful or happy or sad, my openness shifts. It's important to make space for strong feelings in the bedroom. That may mean that we won't have intercourse or it may mean that I am seeking union more actively. Share your emotions. Respect those of your partner. Make space for emotion in the bedroom. The full experience of sexual connection involves all of you – body, mind, heart and spirit. Your emotions need to be honored and so do those of your partner.

Don't Touch Me

I'm also impressed with how much sexual connection (or the lack of it) influences emotion. When one person desires sex and the partner says "No" over and over again, the rejected partner feels justifiably hurt and angry. The partner who says "No" all the time may not appreciate the incredibly strong feelings that are often involved here. There is no getting around this.

I've heard people say "Well, he's just horny. He's using me for sex even though he doesn't care about me." This person has strong feelings that are affecting sexual openness too. Please accept, respect, and share your feelings about sex. It really matters.

Experience

Experience can either enhance openness or take away from it. A history of sexual trauma in childhood or adulthood is a major barrier to openness for many people. Experiences can make you feel insecure because you haven't had many previous sexual partners. Or, you may have had a lot of sexual experience and this might create a lot of openness when you meet someone new. It could go in exactly the opposite direction too. Sex is very individual.

The Older Virgin Man

The movie "The 40-Year-Old Virgin" was a big hit. I know that the movie was a comedy but when I saw it, I felt sad. Feeling that awkward and shut down is a tough situation and there are lots of people out there in exactly the same situation as Steve Carell's character in the movie.

I work with a man who was raised in a very strict interpretation of the Catholic religion. He came to me at only 30 years old. He was raised with a lot of sexual shame. As a teen, he wasn't allowed to see anything provocative on TV or at the movies. He wasn't allowed to spend any time with girls or do any dating, any kind of flirting, or any sexual experimentation at all. It was completely discouraged in his church culture. No dancing, nothing like that.

Dorm Room Drought

When he got to college and he started to experiment a little bit with people, he felt embarrassed and ashamed. He had opportunities to have sex, but he did not take advantage of the opportunities because he felt that sex outside of marriage wasn't in keeping with his values.

By the time he finished college, he still had not had sex. He was starting to feel worried about it. He had a lot of desire, so this wasn't a desire issue. He really didn't have a problem with his body. It wasn't a problem with his environment--he had his own place. He was embarrassed because he'd never had sex.

You're a Virgin?

It became harder and harder for him to find a partner, because now he was embarrassed for being an older virgin and felt so alone in his limited experience.

His lack of experience then affected his emotions. He felt shame, sadness, and embarrassment. His energy around sex was very closed down; he didn't put himself out there as someone desiring sex. It wasn't that he was struggling with fatigue, like some people. His was a barrier to openness based on experience.

No Sexy Vibe

His sexual energy was very withheld. He didn't put out any kind of sexy vibe into the world that somebody else might've picked up. So people who might have hooked him up with a friend or been interested themselves just thought he was asexual, or even gay. No one knew that he was interested.

There's Hope

His case is typical of a situation where experience (even without sexual trauma) has a strong effect on sex today. If this is your life, take heart. This man got over the hump and started accepting himself sexually. He realized that his lack of experience was only a barrier if he let it be. He learned to be fully present in his body. He found a loving relationship with a passionate sexual connection.

Eroticism

Eroticism opens us up to sexual experiences in different ways. When the sex you're being offered is aligned with your eroticism, you become more open in the bedroom.

The Good Stuff

People often feel too tired and busy and stressed because the sex they're having isn't very good. Is your current situation a big zero on your erotic openness scale? It's important to recognize this.

If you don't start talking about what you find erotic, it will be tough to create it in your life.

Tango?

Maybe you'd love to have sex with that amazing tango dancer who performed for President Obama recently in Argentina (google it) but when your partner showed up with a plan for pizza delivery, pop out of a can and "doing it" on a Friday night, your openness just fell flat. Eroticism matters. This doesn't mean that you have to travel to Buenos Aires to have great sex, but maybe signing up for dance lessons at Arthur Murray would be a good start.

Spank Me

Maybe you'd rather "tangle" than tango. BDSM (*Bondage/Discipline/Dominance/Submission/Sadism/Masochism) is a lot more common - and a lot healthier - than many people think. The wonderful thing about the BDSM community (and it's a huge community) is that negotiation and consent is at the core of all erotic power play. The vanilla community could learn a lot about sharing needs, expectations and desires from the kinky crowd. Interested in getting tied up in the bedroom? Check out the resources at the back of the book to find out more.

7 Minutes in Heaven

"I don't have time for sex." I hear this all the time.

When you think about the fact that the average sex experience for American couples is 7-10 minutes in duration and many couples are having sex once a month, (maybe once a week if they're an active couple), that's 10 minutes a week, time 4.5

weeks a month. That's 45 minutes a month having sex. That's not very much time with you consider all the hours we have in any one day.

It's not the time. We may feel too busy, but that's really openness talking. When you feel erotically charged, you will find time.

Stressed to the Max

I get that you're too stressed out for sex right now. Totally get that. That's because by the time you think about all the stuff you need to think about and get all that out of your head somehow and then you manage to process the things with your partner that have been upsetting you, it literally can take forever. Eroticism is way down the list.

Not Again

Maybe the last time you had sex, it didn't work out very well and you don't want that to happen again. You didn't get much out of it. He lost his erection and felt frustrated. You wondered if he just wasn't into you.

Empowerment

Empowerment is a critical piece of sexual openness. When you don't feel at cause in your own life sexually, it's almost impossible to access deep erotic energy. You might love to relinquish control completely as a sub in a dom/sub relationship, but you still stand in a place of your own power even as a sub.

When you don't fully connect with your lived experience of empowerment, it's tough to open up in the bedroom.

CHAPTER NINE

O = Orgasm

> "A word about orgasm, it's dessert,
> not the main course."
>
> Mary Klein, *Sexual Intelligence*

The media and Hollywood are lying to us when they say that orgasm is the only thing that matters during sex and simultaneous orgasm is the only goal. That's just false.

Oh No!

Orgasm is a peak emotional experience, a peak pleasure experience, but not some kind of contest. While orgasm is a positive, wonderful thing for lots of people, some have never fully experienced an orgasm. The stress on these people ruins sex. How ridiculous!

Sometimes these people actually have had an orgasm but because they're expecting to see what happens in the movies, they don't realize it. "Well I haven't ever had an orgasm, because I didn't scream out with pleasure or look like I was going to faint. I guess I just don't have orgasms."

I love orgasm as much as the next person, and orgasm is important but I want you to know that sex is a whole experience of pleasure and not just one peak moment.

When Your Partner Gets Off

When you see your partner getting ready to have an orgasm, how do you react? Are you goal oriented? Are you thinking "I've got to get my partner off" or it (sex) "doesn't count". I hope not. I hope that you're able to be present with your partner without performance expectations.

Let It Be

Giving the woman her "O" has become such a focus that in some situations, if she doesn't orgasm, her partner actually shames her. She's under pressure now. Remember that pressure and stress are the enemies of pleasure. The phenomenon of faking orgasm is born out of this. Enjoy the moment. Communicate with your partner and stick with it to provide pleasure but don't put the pressure on. Let it be. It's all okay.

Skill Set

People don't often have the skills to please their partner sexually. The key here again is communication and negotiating what to do. Women and men both need to tell their partners what they like. Do you like it hard or soft? Do you want more or less lube (or no lube)? Would you like to play with a sex toy? Really communicate. Don't be shy about this. Communicate about what's going well and what isn't.

Speaking of Toys

There are wonderful sex toys on the market. Don't miss the fun. Sex toys are made in all sorts of sizes and shapes. You can buy them in glass, stainless steel or medical grade silicone. You can buy them vibrating or not. There are great online resources at the back of the book where you can find something just right. A couple of tips about your toys:

1. **Watch out for toxic toys**.
   When you are buying a sex toy, make sure it doesn't smell "like a plastic shower curtain". That smell comes from a murky mixture of chemicals that I don't want anywhere near your lovely body. The basic culprit is called phthalate (pronounced "thal-late"). Since sex toys are not regulated by the FDA for use, you need to take special care when you buy yours.

   The resources at the back of the book will direct you to sex shops where the toys are not only hot - they're safe to use directly on your body.

2. **Keep your toys nice and clean**.
   Your sex toys should always be kept clean. Wash them thoroughly with warm, sudsy water after use. You can also use a condom on your sex toy just like you would on a partner.

3. **Enjoy your toy but don't numb up**.
   Stay connected to your body through self touch with your own fingers and touch from your partner. Toys are great but be mindful that overuse of vibrating toys can decrease your sensitivity to other types of touch.

Confidence is Hot

How much do sexual skills matter in bed? Some of my clients are really worried that they don't know how to give a great blow job or go down on a woman with flair.

Speak Up

Sexual skills do matter but what matters more is confidence and communication; that's what's really sexy. Sexual skills are simply a negotiated interaction between people. You show your partner what you like. You use your own hand if your partner is not using it correctly or talk about how your partner is doing oral sex on you. Speak up.

More Teeth?

If your partner is giving you oral sex, give feedback. Faster? Slower? More friction? More suction? More tongue? Less Teeth? Explain to each other what you like and what you don't like and be super honest about it.

What's an Orgasm?

Orgasm is a really important experience for many people, but it's also something that is overly emphasized. Orgasm is a peak pleasure experience. You get to claim it. No one is judging your orgasm. Nobody should tell you that it is or isn't an orgasm. An orgasm doesn't have to wait till the end of your experience. A lot of people think orgasm is where things stop, but sometimes it's where things start.

O's Are in the Brain

It's fascinating to know that orgasm is a central nervous system experience of pleasure. It is stimulated physically in the genitals but actually occurs in the pleasure center of the brain. If you have decided that your "body just isn't built for orgasm" it may surprise you that people who have had spinal cord injuries also experience orgasm even when they have no sensation below the injury area. This is because the orgasmic response of pleasure is perceived in the brain. The brains of these spinal cord injury individuals are intact and able to experience pleasure. In fact, many people develop highly erotic areas above the area of injury. Your ability to experience pleasure as a sexual being is wide-ranging and magical.

Thinking Off

As this book goes to press, there are candidates entering a study at Rutgers University where they will be "thinking off", i.e., having orgasm solely from mental erotic stimulation. As they experience orgasm from only their thoughts, they will be hooked up to brain scanners that will watch the orgasmic pleasure centers in the brain to confirm their orgasmic experiences. Now, that's research!

Multiplication tables

How about multiple orgasms? Do they matter?

There's nothing wrong with multiple orgasms. If you have the goal of having multiple orgasms, once you've reached that goal, you won't know what all the fuss was about.

Multiple orgasms don't matter at all. What matters are multiple moments of being completely present and connected to your partner.

Now that I've said that, you should know that men can have multiple orgasms and so can women, but the number of orgasms you have or your partner has is not the point. The point is connecting and pleasuring each other.

When the train leaves the station too early

I have been working with a married couple in their 20's where orgasm was a problem. He had very significant early ejaculation. It was demoralizing for him and very upsetting and frustrating for her too. Even though they were young, she told him that she wasn't going to have sex anymore because it was so frustrating.

Do Your Exercises... 1 and 2 and 3

Through our coaching, this young man learned how to delay ejaculation using a muscle training program and masturbation. He thought about using a numbing cream on his penis, but decided against it because she didn't want to get numb during sex.

Eventually, he decided to use Prozac to treat his condition. In addition to this sexual concern, he had a history of depression. Prozac has the sexual side effect of delayed ejaculation - perfect for this couple. Once they got the Prozac on board, they had great sex, wonderful connection and increased intimacy.

It was much better. Of course it wasn't perfect. But even those times when he orgasmed too soon, they didn't stop being sexual. There are so many things that a couple can do sexually without an erect penis.

Get Creative

Don't limit yourself to a sexual script. For example, in their case, when he comes too early he uses a nice dildo on her. Instead of limiting themselves during each session, they mix it up. You can do this too. Many couples do the same thing every time they have sex. Don't do this. Be creative.

Get a Dildo

In fact, I recommend that you have a dildo that you enjoy no matter what your situation. Maybe you want something to play with that's small, large, big girth, small girth, glass, metal, vibrating or not vibrating. It doesn't even have to be a penis shape; it could be another shape. There are a lot of choices out there, fantastic choices. You can use them to stimulate any or all of your erotic zones—even the public parts of your body like your neck, hands, arms and feet.

Show Up

It's really important to disconnect the satisfaction of the session from who has an orgasm, and when they orgasmed. It doesn't mean anything. The only thing that matters is fully showing up and sharing pleasure.

It's Not a Performance

That whole piece that the media, Hollywood, and your upbringing have given you is a sense that there's something guiding the action – almost like a script. You start out, somebody says something; that means that maybe you're going to have sex. Then you kiss and there's a French kiss involved. Uh-oh, that means we are going to have sex. Your partner goes up and starts the bathwater; yup - definitely wants sex. Then you start kissing. Your partner gives you oral sex. You give your partner oral sex. Your partner enters you or you enter your partner. Your partner has an orgasm; you have an orgasm. It's done. That's a wrap.

The Sex Script

If you asked most couples to write down the script for what they do when they have sex, it would be exactly the same every single time. No variation. You know what to do. And in some ways that's good, because then you don't get confused. You're on script; you know what's next.

But it can be also boring, and it can cause people to have limitations. It's like "Uh-oh. Well, this thing's over and we aren't going to do it again for a month. It's New Year's Eve and we're talking maybe February 1st before we get around to it again." That's just not a good plan.

So orgasm needs to be disengaged from the whole thing in terms of what happens. You need to welcome variety.

Orgasm and intercourse

A lot of women don't have orgasm with intercourse, and there's no goal around that either. Just let go of feeling like there's some kind of a contest going on, or that somehow people are judging you, or of judging yourself. Any kind of "spectatoring", where you're watching yourself needs to stop. "Oh my gosh, I think my butt looks bad" or "My O face" is not as hot as the people in the movie" or whatever. Just let go of any kind of judgment about your pleasure. They call it pleasure for a reason.

Enjoy it. Enjoy it. Enjoy it.

CHAPTER TEN

M = Mindfulness

> "We all have inherited preconceptions and ideas about sex, which are mostly false and form a screen, or barrier, that separates us from the real power of sex."
>
> Diana Richardson and Michael Richardson,
> *Tantric Sex for Men, Making Love a Meditation.*

At first glance, mindfulness doesn't seem like a sexual topic. It brings to mind quiet meditators or yogi's who look inside themselves to connect with the All That Is and with their own experience of spirituality. They are epitomized by celibate Buddhist monks. It's a wonderful topic but not inherently hot. In fact, by definition it's not hot. It's detached and spiritual.

Hopeless to Hot

Let's take a second look at mindfulness and sex. In truth, mindfulness can take your bedroom from hopeless to hot in a moment. If you and your partner are able to step fully together into a moment, to hold that space of pleasure with complete presence and energetic union, nothing else that we've discussed here will even matter. The room will disappear, time will melt away, your bodies will merge and you will meet in a place of true connection. This is the promise of sexual union. Your life will be transformed in that instant. Like wow. For reals. Definitely hot and definitely spiritual.

Get Your Head in the Game

But there's a big "if" in this promise. That big "if" is keeping you from a transformational sexual connection. Your lack of presence during sex is your number one barrier to true connection.

You must know the old joke about the biggest sex organ being between the ears and not between the legs, right? But, if you're like the rest of us, a lot of the time you end up thinking about everything but sex - even during sex.

Or you might be thinking about sex but you're not being in sex in a way that allows your thoughts to float by like clouds on a Mid-western afternoon, floating high in the sky. You're thinking about your performance, or your physical flaws. You are not being fully present to pleasure.

Running Commentary?

Instead of simply being present, your thoughts consume you. You struggle to connect with your own body. You're overcome with negative self-talk--that running commentary about your thighs or your smell or your erection.

Am I losing it? Is she noticing? Did she come yet? Shit.

You're so worried about how you look, sound and feel that you're not actually seeing or hearing or sensing the moment. Instead of mindful connection and blissful release, you have running snarky commentary going on.

Read All About It

It's your own version of a CNN news flash text running at the bottom of your inner screen that keeps you from truly being present and having the most important, incredible moment of your life. It could be a moment that rocks you to the depth of your soul but instead it looks and feels like this:

Breaking News:

Cock not hard enough tries to enter female not wet enough while seconds tick down before he gets off and they revert back to fighting about sex for another 14-21 days. Updates at eleven.

Think of George Bush

Mental distraction, either intentional (think of George Bush so you won't come) or unintentional (what are you going to get at Costco later today) keeps you from truly connecting. You've always got static on the line.

Costco

One of my clients thinks about her Costco shopping list while she's having sex. They usually do it in the morning right before they go for a big shopping trip and she is distracted with everything she has to buy. She tries to remember to write things down when they're done like the snacks for soccer on Saturday and the cat litter. A great plan for her is to either change the time they have sex or the time they go shopping.

Are You In There?

That kind of mental distraction makes your partner feel like you're not actually in the room. In truth, you really aren't.

Create a Mental Space for Sex

This has to do with your intention to make sex a priority. When you cultivate erotic thoughts during the day, you keep a mental bookmark open for sex all the time. You welcome sex into your mental space.

Taking the parking brake off to allow sex to happen is a mindfulness approach. The cognitive inhibition of sexual activity in both men and women dampens arousal so that we can function in society without getting arrested (usually). Taking off the mental parking brake is important before arousal can happen.

Many people know that they have a strong parking brake on but have no idea where the handle is or how to release it.

Dial in Erotic Thoughts

You'll be able to identify what the parking brake was and how your thoughts might have turned you away from sex. When you are able to change your thoughts a little bit you become open to sex and arousal.

You can consciously remove the parking brake and open yourself up to the natural, pleasurable experience that is sex. Then, show up in the moment, ready to connect mindfully.

That Sounds like too Much Planning

When sex is negotiated, thought about, planned, and even scheduled can it still be erotic, hot and passionate?

When we negotiate and plan for sex some people say "Oh I don't want to have scheduled sex, that's like a duty thing and we put it on the calendar, that's not right. We should just be tearing each other's clothes off on the kitchen table. The only hot sex is Hollywood sex and it looks like people don't have any planning around it at all." Well, actually they do. They're working off of a script all the time. Because it's Hollywood.

Negotiating and scheduling sex means that we are making it a priority. It means that we've gotten ourselves ready. We can cultivate the sense of eroticism and arousal and it can be incredibly hot.

Boring?

Let me ask you this: if somehow you got yourself onto Craig's List and made an agreement with a sexy willing partner would planning for sex be a problem?

What if it went something like this?

Craig's List [your town listed here]
NSA (No Strings Attached) Afternoon Delight Encounter Female looking for Male

Meet me at the Crowne Plaza Hotel on Highway 169 near the off ramp right across from the golf course second floor, room 217.

I'll put the door guard on so that you can let yourself in without a key. I'll be in bed with the lights off and a candle burning.

I brought some tequila in case you want a shot. It will be on the dresser. I can't wait!!

Now, you may find that kind of secret rendezvous offensive, dangerous, or inappropriate, but I doubt you would find the planning boring.

Not.

It's hot. And the people who end up in that hotel room in the middle of the day will be shaking with desire as they enter that room. Planning isn't inherently a buzz kill. It's all in how you show up. Of course if it looks like duty sex and it feels like duty sex, it's not hot.

How can I get out of my head?

You can improve your sex life by taking time to be still and quiet every single day. Meditation practices will allow you to quiet the monkey mind within you to decrease your stress and improve your sex life.

Sex = Really Bad

Negative thoughts about sex affect sexual satisfaction. Where do these thoughts come from? Many people were raised to believe that human sexuality is inherently shameful. These thoughts may be cultural, religious, or related to family dynamics where sex was either seen as something bad, or was never discussed.

Often, the message was "sex is bad and you will not talk about it, think about it, ask about it, do it or want to do it - unless and until you are married to the right person - someone of the opposite sex who is acceptable as an appropriate partner to me, and to your Mom. Any questions?"

But Now it's Really Good

"When you do get married, have wonderful pleasure and let yourself go because now it totally ok, pretty much. Well, not that much but still have fun if you don't act too dirty. Got it?"

The Sex Box

It's no wonder that we are filled with shame when we open the sex box. It's a huge challenge for all of us - even me. Try being me out there explaining what I do. Try being my kid and telling somebody's mom that your mom is a sex coach. Try saying over and over that you don't sleep with your clients.

This stuff is all okay but it's a challenge. The reason it's so confusing is that we don't talk much about sex in our culture. When we do, all sorts of stuff comes out.

Sex Shaming

Sex shaming is the real deal. You've got to deal with it if you're going to make progress designing your pleasure- drenched BED-ROOM life starting now. So call it what it is and move on. When you recognize sex shaming rearing its ugly head, acknowledge its presence, thank it for trying to keep you safe, offer a polite "you gotta go now handshake" and show it the door. Bye bye shame guy. Sayonara.

When Sex Gremlins Show Up

How does mindfulness play into sex? It comes in with every single aspect of sex that we've discussed so far. It has to do with the way we think about sex and what we do with that monkey mind when we're having sex, and whether or not we're able to release ourselves to the pleasure of sex. It affects whether we're allowing ourselves to really create a state of connection with sex, allowing the clouds of thought to float by and not get attached to them during a sexual encounter.

During sex, align yourselves and take a deep breath and watch the thoughts going by, but don't bring them in. Allow yourself to be in the space between the thoughts and find the gap between thoughts and being-ness.

At its best, that's what sex really is - a connection with the pleasure, the pure pleasure of your own body and that sense of being in the gap of gorgeous, energetic, joyous experience, and then finding your partner there too. That is absolutely beautiful sexual connection.

What matters is being truly present and truly connected in the moment, out of your head and into your body and pleasure; the giving and the receiving with your partner.

Tantric sex

There are specific things about mindfulness that are practices. Tantric sex is a type of mindful sex. Now, that doesn't mean to say that you can't have other types of sex that include mindfulness. Mindfulness is just letting go of all of your thoughts while you're in the process of being sexual with your partner.

But tantric sex is specifically designed for that. And, it's great for people who've had the kinds of the struggles we've already talked about, like erectile dysfunction or challenges with early ejaculation. For a woman, having a slower arousal pattern where it takes some time for her to warm up can be nicely addressed by a tantric approach.

Yab Yum

Tantric positions are great for establishing connection. I recommend *Yab-Yum* to people I work with. In a male-female situation, the woman sits on the man's lap, and she crosses her legs behind his buttocks. Then the man, depending on how limber he is, crosses his legs behind her buttocks, or he could have his legs out in a "V." He may or may not have an erection.

Clothes On

Even though they can do this completely clothed, there's an energetic charge between the genitals of a man and a woman. Her left arm goes under his right arm and comes around his back, and her right arm goes over his left arm and goes around his neck.

Eye Gaze

Then they look at each other, eye to eye, and her left eye goes to his left eye, and they then breathe in through their noses and out through their mouths very slowly, allowing energy to flow between their bodies in a circular fashion, coming down into the chest, up into the genitals, and up the back and then out through the mouth again.

There's a circular experience of energy and breath being exchanged between two people and a mindful, meditative state that goes along with that. When you're involved in this, your goal is to allow your mind to completely disappear and to become one in union with your partner.

Transcend

In this position (as well as in other positions) some people experience transcendent sexual connection, where they feel like they are leaving their bodies and sometimes experience orgasm without any sexual touching at all.

Call 911

One of my female clients experienced a transcendental touch free orgasm during a tantric workshop. Her partner was with her in that moment. When he saw her orgasm, he wanted to call 911 because he thought she was having a stroke! Mindfulness-based sexuality can be very powerful.

Sexual Trauma

Mindfulness can bring you incredible pleasure, even without touching. But your mind can also shut down your sexual experience. I worked with a man who had a very significant childhood sexual abuse history. His thoughts about sex as a married man were impacted by the abuse he suffered as a very young child. Even though his molester was caught and punished, thoughts about the abuse stayed with him for years. It was hard for him to get those thoughts out of his head when he made love with his wife.

His job was to release thoughts about his past through work with me and with a professional therapist who had specialized training in that area. If you have experienced sexual trauma as a child or as an adult, seek professional support. There are resources to help you at the back of this book.

Get Your Head in the Game

When you have negative thoughts in your head and you're ready to let them go remind yourself that you are worthy of pleasure and that sex is good for you. It's great for your health, it's great for your sense of wellbeing, it's great for your cognitive ability as you age, and it creates a great relationship.

Part Three
Create Your BEDROOM Blueprint™

Part 3 gives you the practical tools and the personal inspiration to create a BEDROOM Blueprint™ that will help you build the life of your dreams now and in the future.

> "The wise know their days are numbered and act accordingly."
>
> Michael Hyatt & Daniel Harkavy, *Living Forward*

CHAPTER ELEVEN

Your Bedroom Blueprint™ Guide

> "Well, draw yourself a pretty little blueprint and do me a favor and don't show it to me. I like fighting, and I like fucking. I don't care much for thinking."
>
> Cara McKenna, *Willing Victim*

The character in Cara McKenna's erotic novel *Willing Victim* voices the view of most; sex should be spontaneous, hot and unplanned. In fact, the whole idea is that if you have to think about it, just forget it. That's great and all when you're in the heat of your erotic introduction to each other, but what about 20+ years down the road? What then? Give up on passion and connection because you have to think? We're going to try it a different way here.

It's time to dedicate a day to building your BEDROOM Blueprint™. By taking time out of your Too Busy schedule to think about sex, you're going to end up with a hotter, sexier and more passionate relationship than you ever imagined was possible.

I know that this is a significant time commitment for you, but it's very important to create a blueprint of what you want and need in the bedroom so that your life will be happy, healthy, and filled with pleasure. This is a BEDROOM Blueprint™ guide to help you.

Getting Started

Make sure that you block out a day on your calendar to do this very important work. Choose a place where you feel sexy, whole and connected; a place where you feel that you can get in touch with the erotic person inside you.

If you're in a relationship right now, it would be great if you do this exercise together. If you have kids, get a sitter.

- Plan a day with lunch in a romantic restaurant. Find somewhere with beautiful lighting.
- Dress up. If you have the money in your budget, do something special for yourself like a makeover, a blowout, or a mani-pedi.
- If that's not in your budget (or your style,) just do something for yourself so that you feel good in your own skin.
- Feel as sexy as you possibly can - alone or with a special person. Put on something that makes you feel your best.

You want to feel incredibly good about who you are when you do this exercise. Be sure to unplug your phone. Let others know where you are so you can relax, but ask that they not interrupt you as you do the exercises here. Stay upbeat.

This planning experience is inspired by the process advocated by Michael Hyatt and Daniel Harkavy in their wonderful book *Living Forward* (2016).

Creating your BEDROOM Blueprint™ is a practical approach to an area of your life that can seem impossible to solve. Yup! This is a sex productivity process - an important but unusual approach to making your sex life just as good or better than the rest of your life. (Just a thought - after you finish this process, maybe you can jump on over to *Living Forward* and plan out the rest of your life. Use your success in the bedroom to fuel success at work, in your health, and your finances.)

Despite what the wonderful Cara McKenna says, you need to remember that sex is not magic. It can be magical if you use the same techniques that you use to solve all the other challenges you face every day to make it work just right. You can do this.

It's a challenging task, but an important one. If you approach this process with an open and accepting attitude, it will be lots of fun. There are no right or wrong answers here. Your goal is to be honest with yourself about what you truly want. Here we go!

Your First Step

Many people share the fantasy of growing old together as lovers, sitting on a park bench, holding hands together and holding each other. You're going to create a vision of your future self.

Your Park Bench Moment

Imagine yourself as a little old man or a little old woman sitting on a park bench or in a coffee shop or maybe on your own couch in front of a fireplace.

Look down at your hands and see the wrinkles and the age spots.

Ask yourself "Do I have a partner?" If you do, see the veins in your hand as you hold the hand of your partner. As you hold your partner's hand you feel warmth and love. You softly stroke your partner's hand.

Imagine talking with your partner about the wonderful relationship you've had all these years. Imagine how you've felt together, what you've seen together, and what types of adventures you've shared. Take a minute to think about your experiences. Think about your love life. How has it been over the years?

- Remember some of the most incredible sexual moments you've had together. Where are some of the places you've made love?

- Maybe you were in Prague overlooking the Old Town with your foot up on a radiator as people passed by unknowing in the street below.

- Maybe you found your way off the bike path on a sunny day and made love out in the woods.

- Maybe you had gorgeous moments together in your delightful bedroom under the eves with an old oak tree scratching against the window in the middle of a pounding Midwestern storm.

- Maybe you remember making love with the waves crashing outside on vacation in Mexico.

Let your mind wander and envision the incredible moments that you and your partner have experienced together during your incredible lives.

If you don't have a partner right now, just imagine a perfect situation for you--a sexual life where you have felt completely comfortable, fully welcomed, and totally understood.

Now think about how people describe you:

- How alive you seem

- How passionate you seem

- How you show up with so much energy
- How people can't believe your age

Once you have your vision in mind, think about your siblings, your good friends, people you know and people that you've known all along. Envision yourself having many of these friends even now that you are very old.

Your Second Step

- Take out your journal and start to write down what you have envisioned here. Write down all of the details that you've imagined and include them in your journal.
- Try to include specific details about the smells, the sights, the sounds, the memories and the places you've been.
- Write down the things you've done together and how you feel right now as you sit here together.
- Write them all down and make it feel as though you are actually living this moment. (You can use your phone to dictate your vision if you want to instead of writing it.)
- Once you have finished, (if you have a partner right now) read it out loud and share your vision together. Take time to let it sink in.

_____

_____

_____

Your Third Step

Take a moment to think about the seven BEDROOM areas one-by-one:

- BODY
- ENVIRONMENT
- DESIRE
- RELATIONSHIP
- OPENNESS
- ORGASM
- MINDFULNESS

Start with your body.

How does your body feel now that you are old?

- How does it look? What are some of the things about your body that have been helpful all these years?
- What things do you love about your body even now that you're old? What is your body still able to do? Can you dance? Walk?
- Can you still have sex?

What kinds of challenges does your body have now? Have you struggled with your weight? Have you had trouble with your joints or your health? How about your hair? Are you happy with your skin?

In my Park Bench Moment, I will think about how my bedroom body has been for all these years. I will reflect on what has happened. I feel good about it because:

_____

_____

_____

Now that you've completed this process for your body, go through the same process for the remaining six BEDROOM areas. Continue imagining your future self - your Park Bench Moment in each of the BEDROOM areas.

Your future self - Your Park Bench Moment

Write down a few sentences for each area using the questions below:

How does your environment feel now that you are old?

- How does it look? What are some of the things about your environment that have been helpful all these years?
- What things do you love about your environment even now that you're old?
- Do you live in the same place that you live now?

In my Park Bench Moment, I will think about how my bedroom environment has been for all these years. I will reflect on what has happened. I feel good about it because:

_____

_____

_____

How does your desire feel now that you are old?

- How does it feel? What are some of the things about your desire that have been helpful all these years?
- What things do you love about your desire even now that you're old?
- Do you still have desire? If not, when did it disappear in your life?

In my Park Bench Moment, I will think about how my desire has been in the bedroom for all these years. I will reflect on what has happened. I feel good about it because:

_____

_____

_____

How does your relationship feel now that you are old?

- How does it feel? What are some of the things about your relationship that have been helpful all these years?

- What things do you love about your relationship even now that you're old?

- Are you in love?

In my Park Bench Moment, I will think about how my relationship in the bedroom has been for all these years. I will reflect on what has happened. I feel good about it because:

_____

_____

_____

How does your openness feel now that you are old?

- How is your openness now? What are some of the things about your openness that have been helpful all these years?

- What things do you love about your openness even now that you're old?

- Are you open in the bedroom even now?

In my Park Bench Moment, I will think about how my openness in the bedroom has been for all these years. I will reflect on what has happened. I feel good about it because:

_____

_____

_____

How does your orgasm feel now that you are old?

- How is your orgasm? What are some of the things about your orgasm that have been helpful all these years?
- What things do you love about your orgasm even now that you're old?
- Can you still orgasm? Do you?

In my Park Bench Moment, I will think about how my orgasm has been for all these years. I will reflect on what has happened. I feel good about it because:

_____

_____

_____

How does your mindfulness feel now that you are old?

- How does it seem? What are some of the things about your mindfulness that have been helpful all these years?
- What things do you love about your mindfulness even now that you're old?
- Are your thoughts about the bedroom positive?

In my Park Bench Moment, I will think about how my mindfulness in the bedroom has been for all these years. I will reflect on what has happened. I feel good about it because:

_____

_____

_____

When you are finished thinking and writing about each of the seven BEDROOM areas, you'll have a beautiful vision of your happy little old self sitting on the park bench of your future.

Some of the things you might have discovered are places you've explored over the years. Maybe you've visited places like Bali, India, Hawaii or Mexico. Maybe you've lived the life of a mountain biker in Durango Colorado and have scars on your knees to prove it. Maybe you've been a surfer in Ventura, California or a climber on Mount Hood in Oregon.

Your BEDROOM Blueprint™ is the tool you'll use to get from here to there. In order to do that, you need to know where you are right now. Let's dive deep into the seven bedroom areas so that you can make a plan to make that vision a reality.

Ready?

For each of the seven bedroom areas, you'll have a chance to reflect on several questions and write about your answers. Then you'll do an exercise to take you deeper into knowing yourself in that area. Finally, you'll create a BEDROOM Blueprint™ based on what you find out.

We'll start with your body.

BODY

Write in your journal about your body in the bedroom:

Exercise: Sit down with a piece of paper and write down every word you can think of that has anything to do with sex, your sexual body parts, or your partner's sexual body parts. Circle the words you like in green, the words you are OK with in yellow, and the words that you don't like in red. Ask your partner to do the same. Exchange lists. Talk about what you've discovered. Find common language. Make a plan and write about it here:

_____

_____

_____

Now explore your body in the bedroom:

Body Awareness Exercise (for men and women):

For this exercise, you will need:

- A private space with a full length mirror
- Your journal
- Two colored pencils: one red and one green

Set a timer for 15 minutes to do the exercise.

Take off your clothes. Stand in front of the full-length mirror.

Start at the top of your head and notice your body. Say out loud what you like about your body and what you don't like.

Note: If you want to do this exercise with your partner, you are welcome to do so but your partner is only to listen kindly to your words and to make no comments either positive or negative.

Continue from your head to your toes and notice your body, making comments out loud about how you see yourself. Try to see the back of your body too.

When you've scanned and commented on your whole body, take out your journal and your colored pencils. Write down what you've noticed about your body there. For example, "I see my hair has a new haircut, I like that, I don't like my neck, it's sagging," etc.

When you're finished, use your red pencil to circle the negative words you've written about your body and the green pencil to circle the positive words or phrases.

Take a look at what you've written. Breathe in gratitude for your living body today. If your body page shows a lot of red, make a plan to begin releasing body shame. There are resources that will help you do that in the resource section of this book. Just noticing is the first step to becoming whole.

1.   How did you feel when you first started the exercise?

_____

_____

_____

2.   What part of your body was the most pleasing to see and why?

_____

_____

_____

3. What part of your body was the most difficult for you to think about and why?

_____

_____

_____

4. What feelings did you have as you did this exercise?

_____

_____

_____

5. What thoughts did you have as you looked at your body?

_____

_____

_____

6. How have your thoughts and feelings about your body affected your life up until now?

_____

_____

_____

7. How would your life change if you were able to start loving your body fully from now on?

_____

_____

_____

8. How can you start seeing your body with love now and in the future?

_____

_____

_____

9. If you were unable to complete the exercise, what was the reason?

_____

_____

_____

Exploring Your Body Exercise (just for women):

What you will need:

- Privacy
- A hand held mirror
- Your journal
- A pen or pencil

    1. You can do this exercise alone or with a partner.
    2. Take off your clothes and lie down on your back with your legs slightly apart.
    3. Use the mirror to take a look at yourself between your legs.

What do you see? Open your beautiful lips to reveal the moist inner lips and the opening to your vagina.

Can you see your clitoral head?

Can you see the tiny urethral meatus? This is where urine comes out of your body.

Bear down as if you're having a bowel movement and see what that does to your body. You may be able to see your G Spot tissue at the mouth of your vagina when you do this.

Now, apply lubricant to your fingers and touch yourself a little bit. Notice how you like it. Stroke your clitoris and your inner and outer lips.

Feel inside your vagina. Where and how do you like to be touched?

When you are finished touching yourself, write about this experience in your journal.

You may want to create some art to go with this experience.

You may want to draw your genitals in your journal.

Notice your experience and share it if you are comfortable.

_____

_____

_____

ENVIRONMENT

Continue to learn about yourself in the bedroom as you explore the impact of your environment in your life.

Write in your journal about your environment in the bedroom:

1.   How does your environment affect you sexually?

_____

_____

_____

2.   What could you do to make your environment comfortable for being with a partner?

_____

_____

_____

3.   What kind of things get in the way of feeling sexual with your partner in your home?

_____

_____

_____

4.   Where would you love to go to get away?

_____

_____

_____

5.   If you don't have a partner, how does your environment reflect your sexual self now?

_____

_____

_____

6. How would you like your environment to reflect your sexual self in the future?

_____

_____

_____

Now explore your bedroom environment:

Exercise: For this exercise you will need:

- A camera
- Your journal
- Pen or pencil

Set aside 15" for this exercise. Do not clean up your space before you start.

Take your camera to your room. Take at least four photos. Be sure to photograph details. Now, sit down with your phone and a timer. For each of the four photos spend 3 minutes writing about what you see.

Just describe, don't evaluate.

_____

_____

_____

_____

_____

_____

Now reflect on anything that you know of that is often there but that doesn't show in the photos.

- Do you usually have a dog sleeping between you in the bed?
- Do you have kids sleeping with you?
- Do you have privacy in general?
- Do you have other environmental problems in your room?

Complete writing about the current state of your room in your journal. Decide on five things that you can do to make your environment sexier and more relaxing this week.

_____

_____

_____

Continue to learn about yourself in the bedroom as you explore the impact of desire in your life.

DESIRE

Write in your journal about your experience of desire in the bedroom:

1. How do you feel when your partner desires you?

_____

_____

_____

2. How does your partner feel about your desire?

_____

_____

_____

3. What kinds of things would help you feel more desire?

_____

_____

_____

4. What kinds of things would help your partner feel more desire?

_____

_____

_____

5. How has desire been difficult in your life?

_____

_____

_____

6. If you don't have a partner, how do you experience desire in your life now?

_____

_____

_____

7. How would you like to experience desire?

_____

_____

_____

Now explore your desire in the bedroom:

1.   Take out a piece of paper and set the timer to 5 minutes.

2.   Sit quietly in your chair, taking deep breaths and relaxing.

3.   After a few minutes of letting yourself ground into your seat, let your mind wander to a time when you felt sexual desire.

4.   Let yourself feel as though you are in that situation now. Imagine feeling the desire until the timer goes off.

5.   Spend a few minutes writing about your experience:

What did you feel?

_____

_____

_____

Where did you feel it?

_____

_____

_____

What emotions did you have about your feeling of desire?

_____

_____

_____

What were your thoughts?

_____

_____

_____

In what ways can you welcome feelings of desire into your life right now?

_____

_____

_____

How would you describe this experience to your partner (or a potential partner)?

_____

_____

_____

RELATIONSHIP

Continue to learn about yourself in the bedroom as you explore the impact of relationship in your life.

Write in your journal about your relationship in the bedroom:

1. How has your relationship been affected by sex?

_____

_____

_____

2. How comfortable are you with your couple sexual style
    (frequency, who initiates, when and where you make love)?

    _____

    _____

    _____

3. How would your couple sexual style look if it were just right
    for you now?

    _____

    _____

    _____

4. How about for your partner?

    _____

    _____

    _____

5. If you don't have a partner, what would a perfect partner
    look, sound and feel like?

    _____

    _____

    _____

6. What could you do to find that person right now?

    _____

    _____

    _____

Have a partner now? Explore your relationship in the bedroom:

Take out 2 pieces of paper. Make an agreement to communicate with kindness as you do this exercise.

Write out the script for a typical sexual encounter between you.

When you're finished, compare notes.

How similar are they?

Ask each other if the way you typically make love is what you'd like to have happen.

If there's something you'd both like to change, discuss a way to do that. Make sure that this is done with complete kindness. For example, if the man is struggling with erectile dysfunction or the woman is having issues with desire or orgasm, emphasize connection and love in your discussion.

Support each other as you make a plan to re-write your script. Or, celebrate the fact that you both like it just the way it is.

Note: I often get asked: "What if my partner wants to do something sexual that's not okay with me? Maybe it's totally outside of my comfort zone."

Well, it's my opinion that it's better to get the cards out on the table when it comes to sex. I think that it's better to know today and see what you can do to come to some agreement that respects the needs and wishes of everyone involved. You'll have to decide for yourself if you want to know the truth of what your partner is thinking.

OPENNESS

Continue to learn about yourself in the bedroom as you explore the impact of your openness in your life.

Write in your journal about your openness in the bedroom:

1. How have emotions affected your sexual relationship?

   _____

   _____

   _____

2. How has your experience influenced you sexually?

   _____

   _____

   _____

3. How does your energy influence your sexual connection with your partner?

   _____

   _____

   _____

4. If you don't have a partner, how would you like to experience sexual openness in the future?

   _____

   _____

   _____

5. How is eroticism (or the lack of it) affecting your openness to sex?

_____

_____

_____

6. How is your sense of being in charge of your own sexual life--your empowerment--influencing your openness?

_____

_____

_____

Now explore your openness in the bedroom:

Take out a piece of paper.

Write about a time when you experienced something sexual that you really enjoyed. It doesn't have to be anything blatantly sexual. Anything that comes to mind will work:

_____

_____

_____

Describe how you felt, what you saw, what you heard, what you were wearing.

_____

_____

_____

Share your thoughts with a partner if you have a partner.

If you are unable to recall a positive sexual experience, imagine something pleasant and sexual. It doesn't have to be really sexual--it could be as simple as a kiss. Write down what you imagine happening, what you think you would feel, see, hear.

Share with a partner or with someone you trust.

_____

_____

_____

ORGASM

Continue to learn about yourself in the bedroom as you explore the impact of orgasm in your life.

Write in your journal about your orgasm in the bedroom:

1. How do you feel about your sexual responsiveness?

_____

_____

_____

2. If you have a partner, how does your partner feel about your sexual responsiveness?

_____

_____

_____

3. If you have a partner, how do you feel about your partner's sexual responsiveness?

_____

_____

_____

Now explore your orgasm in the bedroom:

Find a quiet private place.

Take some deep breaths and give yourself permission to experience pleasure.

Use your hands to explore your body, touching yourself in a way that feels pleasant.

Learn about the sensations your body feels as you touch yourself.

Spend at least 5 minutes touching.

If you are someone who has a self-cultivation (masturbation) practice, expand your self-awareness by learning new things about your body. Extend the time frame.

If you are new to self-cultivation, take this exercise slowly. Dismiss any self-shaming thoughts.

Reflect on the exercise when you are finished.

If you have experienced self-shaming thoughts, review where they might be coming from. Love yourself.

Write about your experience for 3 minutes:

_____

_____

_____

MINDFULNESS

Continue to learn about yourself in the bedroom as you explore the impact of mindfulness in your life.

Write in your journal about your mindfulness in the bedroom:

1. How does your mind affect your sexuality?

    _____

    _____

    _____

2. How do your thoughts affect your relationship with your partner?

    _____

    _____

    _____

3. If you don't have a partner, how do your thoughts affect you as you seek a partner?

    _____

    _____

    _____

4. What would it look like if you created a mindfulness practice for your sexuality?

    _____

    _____

    _____

Now explore your mindfulness in the bedroom:

Sit quietly in a comfortable place.

Take several deep breaths in through your nose and let them out through your mouth.

Allow your mind to wander to your last sexual experience.

Go into the experience fully, recalling the sensations you had at the time. Recall the surroundings, the smells, sights and sounds that accompanied the experience.

Become fully present to the experience, dismissing any thoughts that intrude.

Stay in this moment, allowing it to flow through you.

Open your eyes and reflect on your experience.

If you were flooded with distracting thoughts during the exercise, make note of this quietly to yourself.

The next time you are in a sexual experience, try to be fully present in this way.

Write for 3 minutes about the experience:

_____

_____

_____

_____

_____

Your Final Steps

1.   Create an action item for each area of bedroom.

Now notice the gaps between the current you and the Park Bench You in each area. Decide on which gaps you want to address now and which you'll wait on.

For example, maybe in your vision you've lived and worked in a tropical place like Costa Rica. You had an incredible experience together there--exploring, eating great organic food, learning Spanish, reading and writing together. You made love in a beautiful villa on a hill overlooking the Pacific Ocean every morning when you woke up. It was complete magic.

But for right now, you're raising twin baby girls. You're having trouble finding time to have sex even every week.

So in the area of environment, you see a gap and vow to fill it in the future. For now, you download some Costa Rican music, hang gauzy fabric from the ceiling in your room with push pins, light candles that remind you of the tropics and read sexy stories about Costa Rica as a soft breeze comes in the window and the babies nap. Ahhh peace.

Get it? An action item is something you can do today that will move the current you closer to the Y-O-U you're imagining sitting on that park bench. Your action item is designed to close the gap between what's happening now and what you want to see happen in the future.

Your BEDROOM Blueprint™ Action Items:

Body:

_____

_____

_____

Environment:

_____

_____

_____

Desire:

_____

_____

_____

Relationship:

_____

_____

_____

Openness:

_____

_____

_____

Orgasm:

_____

_____

_____

Mindfulness:

_____

_____

_____

2.   **Create a statement of affirmation in each area of BEDROOM.**

One of the ways that you can move your life closer to the life of your dreams is to create affirmations. Write your affirmations as if you have already experienced the change you are envisioning.

For example, an affirmation statement for BODY might be: "I am strong and limber. I have great balance. I love to dance." There are examples of affirmations for each BEDROOM area in the next chapter. Check them out and see if something feels right for you today.

Your Bedroom Blueprint™ Affirmations:

Body:

_____

_____

_____

Environment:

_____

_____

_____

Desire:

_____

_____

_____

Relationship:

_____

_____

_____

Openness:

_____

_____

_____

Orgasm:

_____

_____

_____

Mindfulness:

_____

_____

_____

Imagine the old you reacting to these action items and affirmations. Will the Park Bench You feel good about what you're saying and doing? Will the Y-O-U of the future be well-served if you begin this BEDROOM transformation today?

To begin to create your own BEDROOM Blueprint™ visit
http://janeguyn.com/startthepath

CHAPTER TWELVE

Your BEDROOM Affirmations

> "I want to get old gracefully. I want to have good posture. I want to be healthy and be an example to my children."
>
> Sting

The power of words to create your reality can't be over emphasized. Neuroscientists confirm that the brain doesn't know the difference between what you tell yourself about your life and what is actually happening. Think about some time that you "got worked up" about something trivial. If you're like most people, your physical response to an imagined threat was as great as it would have been to something very threatening.

The opposite is also true. When you tell yourself through your words that everything is going well, your brain and your body respond accordingly.

This is where positive affirmations come in. And what could be more fun than writing positive affirmations about S-E-X?

And so, let's get to the good stuff - affirmations in the BEDROOM! Below you will find affirmations for each of the seven BEDROOM areas. You are welcome to use these affirmations in your BEDROOM Blueprint™. Or, of course you can write an affirmation of your own for each of the seven BEDROOM areas.

BODY BEDROOM Affirmations

I am lean, limber and strong enough for great sex.

My skin is smooth and sexy, making me a wonderful sex partner.

I look delicious naked.

I am fit and conditioned--ready for sex.

My body responds to my partner beautifully.

I am comfortable with who I am in my own skin.

My genitals are just right.

ENVIRONMENT BEDROOM Affirmations

My room is bathed in sexy, warm light.

My sheets are clean and smooth.

My room smells fresh and sexy.

The temperature is perfect on my skin and makes me feel warm and aroused.

I am relaxed and aroused when I walk in the door of my bedroom.

I love the feeling of lying down in bed with my partner.

DESIRE BEDROOM Affirmations

I feel myself getting turned on when I kiss my partner.

My desire comes over me in waves.

I am surprised at how my desire for my partner is growing every day.

I feel relaxed and comfortable about my desire.

I know how to get turned on when I want to.

I feel confident that I can have a great time in bed.

RELATIONSHIP BEDROOM Affirmations

I am happy in my relationship.

I feel confident that we are creating a life that fits my needs.

My partner responds to me in a way that feels great.

I have a partner in my life who is just right for me.

My partner listens to me.

I feel that my partner thinks I am wonderful.

My partner is always well groomed before sex.

We balance our sex acts--giving and receiving.

I am comfortable asking for what I need from my partner.

We are creating a life that feels good for us both.

OPENNESS BEDROOM Affirmations

I have enough energy to connect in the bedroom with my partner.

My feelings about sex are open and welcoming.

My sexual experiences help me to feel great in the bedroom.

I am empowered in the bedroom; I make my own choices and feel good about it.

My erotic life is a great fit for me.

I am open to sexual connection with my partner.

ORGASM BEDROOM Affirmations

I love how I orgasm.

I feel great about my partner's orgasms.

I am confident in my orgasm.

I do not feel pressured to orgasm in a particular way.

I feel wonderful after I orgasm.

I am able to orgasm with ease.

MINDFULNESS BEDROOM Affirmations

My mind is clear for sex.

I think about sex in a positive way.

I am able to use my thoughts about sex to get ready.

When I have sex, I am present and undistracted.

I use mindfulness to build my sexual connection.

I am aware of my spiritual union during sex.

Just Like Magic?

Once you have decided on 7 affirmations (one for each BED-ROOM area) use them to create the reality you seek. Speak them aloud as if they were already true in your life. Watch the magic happen.

CHAPTER THIRTEEN

Dave and Susie's BEDROOM Blueprint™

Their BEDROOM Blueprint™ Story

Susan (30) and Dave (31) are the lucky parents of darling eight-month-old baby girl Emily. They've been in love for five years and married for three. During the pregnancy, Susan swam in the YMCA pool five days a week and ate well. Still, changes in her body really bothered her after Emily was born. She was horrified with the red, angry looking stretch marks on her tummy at the end of her pregnancy. She put organic coconut oil on her tummy all along in hopes that she'd be one of the lucky ones with a great postpartum bikini body. When those stretch marks showed up during her 35th week, Susan's heart sank.

Dave reassured her that the stretch marks didn't matter at all, but every time Susan saw herself in the mirror after the baby was born, she would tear up. She was disgusted. Sometimes, she saw Dave watching porn on his iPad. This made her feel even worse. The women he watched had perfect bodies and she felt incredibly inadequate about herself when she knew Dave had been watching, no matter how much he told her he thought she was beautiful.

Before the baby, Susan had been an avid yoga participant. She went to yoga during her pregnancy, but as she got bigger yoga got difficult for her. She developed back strain toward the end of her pregnancy and eventually had to quit altogether.

Susan was a great mom. She ate only organic foods and nursed Emily on demand. It took a little while to get started (her nipples cracked and bled at first) but soon they were in a smooth mom-baby groove and Susan loved the bonding experience.

Dave was a very supportive husband and father throughout her pregnancy. They were both very happy when she found out that after only two months of trying she had a positive pregnancy test. During the pregnancy, their sex life actually improved. Susan was very aroused starting in her second trimester. (The first trimester was fairly challenging due to nausea and vomiting.) Dave was encouraged about this. He had lots of friends who'd complained about sex after kids and he was really hoping that he and Susan would beat the odds on this one.

But after Emily's birth, Dave started to feel concerned. Initially, Susan was warm and welcoming to him. Even when she first got home from the hospital, she actively encouraged him to hold her and kiss her. They followed doctor's orders and abstained from sex for the first 6 weeks. When he was able to enter her beautiful body again, Dave felt that he was finally home. They talked a little bit about it later. Susan told him that she didn't really like sex those first few times. In fact, she said that it hurt a lot at first.

He didn't understand why that would be. She'd delivered a 7-pound baby through her vagina. How could his penis cause her pain? The more they had sex, however, the better she liked it. She wasn't really as into it as she'd been before baby, but attributed that to the fact that she was tired from all the nursing. He was actually looking forward to the day when she went back to her full time job. Then things would be back to normal. Wouldn't they?

But after Susan went back to work, things didn't get better at all. Susan stepped right back into her HR role at work. She worked extra hard on team projects and deliverables so that no one could say that somehow her capacity had been diminished by her new role as mom. At home, things got tense. Dave's expectation that things would be "normal" was not born out. He started to feel incredibly rejected by Susan.

He didn't want to admit it but he was starting to resent baby Emily and her invasive relationship with his beautiful wife. They seldom made love anymore, even on those rare date nights when they got a sitter and went out to dinner. Susan always seemed to fall asleep before he could get things closed up downstairs and climb into bed. He felt angry, hurt, isolated and guilty.

What BEDROOM areas are impacting this young, hard-working couple?

Their BEDROOM Blueprint™ Barriers

BODY: Susan is feeling out of touch with her body. It's hard for her to feel sexual when she's struggling with body shame.

ENVIRONMENT: The couple has no privacy. Baby sleeps in the bedroom in a small crib. Even though Dave doesn't mind having sex with Emily in the room, Susan is very aware of Emily's presence. They are not finding a good time for sex.

DESIRE: Susan's desire has been muted by a combination of things including the pregnancy and birth hormones. Dave is feeling intense desire. He is feeling aroused every day. He feels rejected.

RELATIONSHIP: They are fighting over things totally unrelated to sex. He is starting to wonder if she was ever really a sexual person in the past. She is feeling attacked and put down. He is stonewalling her when she won't have sex with him. Their communication is very tense.

OPENNESS: Susan's sexual energy is at an all-time low. She feels like she never gets a minute to herself. Even going to the bathroom alone is a luxury. Dave is really upset because of his experience hearing guys talk about sexless marriages after baby arrives. They are both feeling hurt and misunderstood. They are not sharing erotic thoughts at all.

ORGASM: Susan has had several great orgasms since the baby but she often is too tired to even go there. Dave is upset because he orgasms way too fast. He always had a little problem with being early, but this is getting ridiculous.

MINDFULNESS: Both Dave and Susan are incredibly distracted while making love. She thinks he's looking at her stretch marks when he gives her oral sex. He thinks she's criticizing him when he enters her. He wonders if she is into someone at work. She hates catching a glimpse of herself in the mirror over her dresser. Neither of them is really present during sex.

Their BEDROOM Blueprint™ Action Items

Dave and Susie came up with this great list of things to do to move their relationship closer to what they are hoping for in their Park Bench Moment.

Body:

- Do partner yoga together
- Massage (exchange massages to save money)
- Healthy diet
- Make time for exercise
- Walk in the neighborhood with baby
- Update wardrobe
- Drink plenty of water
- Learn about hormonal changes
- Organic coconut oil to skin, labia, vagina

Body Affirmation: We are strong, limber, and fit. We take care of our bodies. We accept our perfect imperfections with grace and love.

Environment:

- Sexy lighting
- New cotton sheets
- Get a sitter (exchange with a friend to save money) meet at home for lunch sex
- Put baby in the car seat and make out in the front seat

Environment Affirmation: We create a gorgeous sex nest filled with scents, sounds and sexy things. Our linens are clean and smooth. We treat our room as an oasis without electronics.

Desire:

- Spend enough time for her to warm up
- Kissing with no sexual expectations
- Touch the hands, face & feet
- Read erotic stories out loud
- Take sex slowly

Desire Affirmation: We realize that our desire for each other is something that can't be forced. We hold space for desire with kindness and patience. When our desire is uneven, we take it slowly so that we both feel respected. We build desire during the day little by little.

Relationship:

- Schedule family meeting time to discuss conflict
- Journal about concerns
- Be as kind as possible during times of stress
- Get support as people and parents
- Hang out with friends

Relationship Affirmation: We are kind and polite. We create ritual to nurture our connection.

Openness:

- Put sex on the calendar
- Stay in the present
- Make a commitment to getting naked alone no less than every two weeks

- Create an erotic journal
- Record turns ons (share it)
- Reject the negative comments of others
- Keep your erotic energy within the relationship

Openness Affirmation: We keep our erotic energy circulating within our own relationship. We nurture energy for sex by sleeping enough.

Orgasm:
- Masturbate
- Take time for orgasm but don't be pressured
- Let orgasm "ring" afterwards to get the full benefit
- Don't always orgasm in the same order (switch it up)

Mindfulness:
- Meditate
- Release thoughts of shame during sex or about sex
- Cultivate erotic thoughts during the day
- Read erotica
- Reach out for help if having (obsessively) negative thoughts about sex

Mindfulness Affirmation: Our minds are clear for sex.

Nice and easy

Once Dave and Susie had a BEDROOM Blueprint™ that made sense for both of them, they were able to make plans together without unspoken expectations and hurt feelings. What could be easier than that?

CHAPTER FOURTEEN

Conclusion: This is Your Life

> "One of the most universally sexy traits in a person is their confidence."
> — Amy Jo Goddard, *Woman on Fire*

You did it!

You spent a day getting comfortable in your own skin, feeling sexy, connecting with your inner voice, doing expansive exercises, and writing bunches of important notes into either this book or your personal journal.

Congratulations! You are well on your way to an amazing sexual experience--one that deeply resonates with who you truly are today.

You've made great strides today, but this process isn't actually over yet.

Releasing Shame

You've released lots of shame about sex during your personal exploration exercises. Even if you were not consciously aware of shame being released, the act of spending time in truth with your body, space, desire, relationship, openness, orgasm and mindfulness has given you the opportunity to create a bedroom life that works for you.

Now, if you haven't done so already, it's time to share your truth with your partner. If you decide to do the BEDROOM Blueprint™ planning process as a couple you've already done the sharing. If not, now's a great time. Or, you can decide to keep your thoughts and feelings to yourself completely. There is no right answer here.

Show and Tell?

Want to share? Ask for gentleness in the listening. Make sure that you let your partner know how vulnerable you feel sharing your experience.

Update It

The key piece is to keep re-visiting your BEDROOM Blueprint™ so that it stays current for you.

Hang on to the old ones. It will be fun to look back at them as you get older. You'll see changes. Some of the changes will make sex lots easier. Some of them may make it impossible for a time. But, as you see sex in the context of your dynamic life, you'll connect with your personal ability to create and recreate a bedroom life that works.

You don't have to tell your partner every detail of your blueprint right now if you don't want to. It's your private document. Really, it's a key to your deepest heart. Our sexual selves live very deeply within us, so while this looks and sounds like other visioning and goal setting processes, because it's about your sexual self, make sure that you feel comfortable sharing on a deep level before you open your heart in this way.

Hopefully your partner will open up to you, too. If that happens, you'll have an opportunity to share something very special. But even if neither of you chooses to share what you've discovered about yourselves right now, you have the opportunity to do that later when you're both ready. The real work is in looking deep within yourself and honestly seeing what you want, need and desire.

It's a Tough Topic

Congratulations on even "going there."

Sex is a topic that has confused, intimidated and overwhelmed people for decades, centuries, and likely millennia. The magical nature of sex as it's portrayed in Hollywood and in the media plus the way we're taught about sex is often more than just confusing. It is often embarrassing and drenched in shame.

Frankly, sex is fabulous. It's not really all that complicated to deconstruct. Until you add the shame bit. Then it gets dicey.

Maybe a Sex Coach? (Go Team!)

Have you've done your work and still don't know quite what to do next? Does the whole thing sounds great but overwhelming? Maybe you've got a Professional Sex Coach or an AASECT certified sex professional to help you.

Professional Sex Coaching is a new field that's taking hold across the globe. Certified Professional Sex Coaches have extensive education about sexuality that puts them in a position to help people who are struggling with sexual issues. There are resources at the back of the book to help you find the help you need,

Reach out for support so that you can stay on the path to your own bedroom breakthrough.

You've Got the Power

It's up to you to create what you want in your real life. When you enter into the decision-making process about sex with a sense of personal power, you come alive. Along with your intuition, energy, emotions and the things you know about yourself at the deepest level, you'll build something lasting.

Use this practical approach to create a life for yourself that's filled with the type of sexual experience that authentically suits you. You have this information at your fingertips right here for now and for the future. Leave sexual shame behind and claim something authentic and true for yourself.

Welcome to empowered pleasure starting today and lasting until that last beautiful day on that last sweet park bench. I wish you the accepting, loving, welcoming, warmth that you so deeply deserve. Step up to the banquet of the bedroom, your true birthright.

It's your turn.

Books to Support Your Journey

Bass, E., & Davis, L. (1988). *The courage to heal: A guide for women survivors of child sexual abuse.* New York: Perennial Library.

Brame, G. G., Brame, W. D., & Jacobs, J. (1996). *Different loving: The world of sexual dominance and submission.* New York: Villard.

Britton, Patti. (2005). *The art of sex coaching: Expanding your practice.* New York: Norton.

Chapman, G. D. (1995). *The 5 love languages: The secret to love that lasts.*

Charles, A. (2011). *The sexual practices of Quodoushka: Teachings from the Nagual tradition.* Rochester, VT: Destiny Books.

Easton, D., & Hardy, J. W. (2009). *The ethical slut: A practical guide to polyamory, open relationships & other adventures.* NY, NY: Celestial Arts.

Goddard, A. J. (2015.). *Woman on fire: 9 elements to wake up your erotic energy, personal power, and sexual intelligence.*

Gottman, J. M., & DeClaire, J. (2001). *The relationship cure: A five-step guide for building better connections with family, friends, and lovers.* New York: Crown.

Hyatt, M. S., & Harkavy, D. (2016). *Living forward: A proven plan to stop drifting and get the life you want.*

Joannides, P. (2009). *Guide to getting it on: For adults of all ages.* Waldport, OR: Goofy

Katz, A. (2009). *Woman cancer sex.*

Keesling, B. (2006). *Sexual healing: The completest guide to overcoming common sexual problems.* Alameda CA: Hunter House.

Klein, M. (2012). *Sexual intelligence: What we really want from sex-- and how to get it.* New York: HarperOne.

Love, P., & Stosny, S. (2007). *How to improve your marriage without talking about it: Finding love beyond words.* New York: Broadway Books.

McCarthy, B. W., & McCarthy, E. J. (2003). *Rekindling desire: A step-by- step program to help low-sex and no-sex marriages.* New York: Brunner-Routledge.

McKenna, C. (2010). Willing Victim. Received from: www.goodreads.com/book/show/8812286-willing-victim

Mintz, L. B. (2009). *A tired woman's guide to passionate sex: Reclaim your desire and reignite your relationship.* Avon, MA: Adams Media.

Morin, J. (1995). *The erotic mind: Unlocking the inner sources of sexual passion and fulfillment.* New York: HarperCollins.

Nagoski, E. (2015). *Come as you are: The surprising new science that will transform your sex life.*

Ogden, G. (2008). *The return of desire: A guide to rediscovering your sexual passion.* Boston: Trumpeter.

Paget, L. (2005). *Orgasms: How to have them, give them, and keep them coming.* New York: Broadway Books.

Perel, E. (2007). *Mating in captivity: Unlocking erotic intelligence.* New York: Harper.

Richardson, D., & Richardson, M. (2010). *Tantric sex for men: Making love a meditation.* Rochester, VT: Destiny Books.

Ryan, C., & Jethá, C. (2011). *Sex at dawn: How we mate, why we stray, and what it means for modern relationships*. New York, NY: Harper.

Slim, P. (2013). *Body of work: Finding the thread that ties your story together*. NY, NY: Random House.

Sundahl, D. (2003). *Female ejaculation and the G-spot*. Alameda, CA: Hunter House.

Wolf, N. (2012). *Vagina: A new biography*. New York, NY.: Ecco.

Other Important Resources to Help You

To apply for a complimentary BEDROOM Breakthrough™ Discovery Session with me:

http://janeguyn.com/

To find a sex coach:

http://worldassociationofsexcoaches.org/

For understanding the internal clitoris as you never have (fantastic video by Betty Dodson)

http://afterdinnerparty.com/the-clitoris/

For Jade Egg and yoni empowerment workshops:

https://www.kimrosekeller.com

For fantastic illustrations of the clitoris in poster form:

http://www.brightfire.com.au/shop/the-illustrated-clitoris/

For Wedges and other bedroom accessories:

https://www.liberator.com/

For Vaginal Restoration without hormones:

http://www.olgassecret.com/

For essential oils:

https://www.youngliving.com/en_US

For non-toxic sex toys and other erotic gifts:

Good Vibrations: http://www.goodvibes.com/s

Love Revolution: http://loveashland.com/

Smitten Kitten: https://www.smittenkittenonline.com/

She Bop: http://www.sheboptheshop.com/

To learn more about female ejaculation from Deborah Sundahl:

http://isismedia.org/webinars/

To learn more about male ejaculation control and/or to have multiple orgasms:

http://www.climaxwell.com/

For a list of recent Feminist Porn Award Winners:

http://www.feministpornawards.com/

For information from The Mayo Clinic about the causes of painful sex:

http://www.mayoclinic.org/diseases-conditions/painful-intercourse/basics/causes/con-20033293

For information about Pelvic Floor Physical Therapy:

http://www.wildfeminine.com/

For information about sexual aversion:

https://sexualmed.org/known-issues/sexual-aversion/

For detailed information about sexual response models:

https://www.arhp.org/publications-and-resources/clinical-fact-sheets/female-sexual-response

To find an AASECT certified sex therapist:

https://www.aasect.org/

For training to become a Certified Professional Sex Coach:

SexCoachU: http://www.sexcoachu.com/

For getting in touch with what happens when your ignore sex as an issue in your relationship

https://www.reddit.com/r/DeadBedrooms

About the Author

Jane Guyn PhD, RN studied nursing and public health at UCLA. She then completed a training program and worked as a family planning nurse practitioner before moving to distant lands for many years.

Jane is one of the first Professional Sex Coaches in the US with a certificate from the internationally respected SexCoachU and a PhD in Human Sexuality from the Institute for the Advanced Study of Human Sexuality in San Francisco. She is a certified Core Energy coach.

Dr. Guyn coaches individuals and couples using her proprietary BEDROOM Breakthrough™ Solution. She also runs interactive trainings virtually and in person. She lives in Portland, Oregon where her house is filled with lots of wonderful kids and way too many pets. You can find her at www.janeguyn.com.

Made in the USA
Columbia, SC
10 June 2017